Acupressure

Acupressure: Clinical Applications in Musculo-skeletal Conditions

John R. Cross
Dr.Ac MCSP SRP MBAcC MRSH

With a Foreword by James L. Oschman PhD

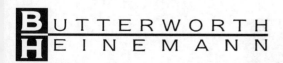

OXFORD AUCKLAND BOSTON JOHANNESBURG MELBOURNE NEW DELHI

Butterworth-Heinemann
Linacre House, Jordan Hill, Oxford OX2 8DP
225 Wildwood Avenue, Woburn, MA 01801-2041
A division of Reed Educational and Professional Publishing Ltd

ℛ   A member of the Reed Elsevier plc group

First published 2000

British Library Cataloguing in Publication Data
Cross, John R.
    Acupressure : clinical applications in musculoskeletal conditions
    1 Acupressure   2 Musculoskeletal system – Diseases –
    Alternative treatment
    I. Title
    615.8'22

ISBN 0 7506 4054 5

Library of Congress Cataloguing in Publication Data
A catalogue record for this book is available from the Library of Congress

ISBN 0 7506 4054 5

Composition by Scribe Design, Gillingham, Kent
Printed and bound by MPG Books Ltd, Bodmin, Cornwall

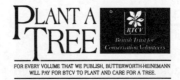

Contents

Foreword

Acupressure: Clinical Applications in Musculo-skeletal Conditions, by John R. Cross, comes at an opportune time, as it embodies and reinforces tremendously exciting trends taking place in health care worldwide. Therapists from diverse disciplines are talking to each other: energy and touch are major topics of the conversation. And biomedical researchers are joining in the discussions. New vistas open up when disciplines that have been kept apart for historical or territorial reasons begin to communicate about theory and method.

In spite of his obvious dedication to the acupressure approach, Cross focuses on what acupressure can contribute as an adjunct to other therapies. Hence his work has direct application for hands-on therapists of every tradition.

So this is not just a book about acupressure. Cross has distilled for us some of the best methods from a range of therapies, as well as his insights from successfully treating thousands of patients presenting a wide variety of problems. This is the opposite of 'staking out a territory to be defended'. Seldom does one find a text that shows such a depth of understanding of allied methods, their history, their strengths and pitfalls and how their best features can be integrated for the benefit of the suffering patient.

Cross has no quarrel with conventional methods: surgery, braces, splints, slings, heat, cold, ultrasound and so on, when they are indicated. Instead, he shows how acupressure can facilitate post-operative and post-trauma healing; he tells us when not to use acupressure – and when it is essential to delay its application. As a result, we have a most valuable text for virtually any hands-on or movement therapist who wishes to extend the range of his or her skills.

Here you will find very practical advice on:

* diagnosis
* what both you and your patient are likely to feel
* optimal treatment sequences
* working away from an area that cannot be touched
* the importance of correct 'firstaid' for certain injuries
* when a treatment should be repeated
* what questions to ask the patient
* how to diagnose from body language, posture and voice tone
* when to use gentle touch or even no touch
* when to be bold.

There are also suggestions on when to warn the patient that a procedure will be painful but worth it for the benefits that will follow. You will find insightful descriptions of the biomechanical origins of common musculoskeletal problems, and how to use a patient's energy system instead of your own to effect a treatment.

Acupressure also comes at a time when science is revealing precisely why energy therapies are so successful. For cells to cooperate in the healing process, defence against disease, or any other collective or cooperative endeavor, they must communicate with each other.

Adjacent cells readily talk to one another via well known couplings and bridges (e.g. desmosomes and gap junctions) spanning the tiny spaces between neighbours. But broader, system-wide communications must go through proper channels, and evidence from a variety of sources shows that these correspond to the acupuncture meridians. Trauma can close down essential flows. When information streams are congested or disorganized, healing proceeds at a snail's pace, if at all. *Acupressure* shows us how to diagnose discontinuity and restore the vital flows.

Cells communicate in quiet and private 'whispers' (research of W. Ross Adey). Hence very small signals, such as those introduced by touch, or projected from a therapist during 'hands-off' treatments, are ideal to initiate healing. The homeopathic principles of 'less is more' and 'small is powerful' are equally important to the language of touch. The reason for this is that living systems routinely amplify tiny signals to produce large effects (see the 1994 Nobel lecture for Physiology or Medicine).

In *Acupressure*, Cross emphasizes natural methods, gentle touch or even no touch, waiting for things to happen rather than forcing. These approaches are consistent with current biomedical research worldwide showing how little energy the body actually requires to trigger a beneficial effect, to 'jump-start' the healing process. To speak the 'language of the cell' signals must be of low intensity and of the appropriate frequency, and there is no better source than the hands of the experienced and well-intentioned therapist.

Pioneers are constantly standing on the shoulders of their teachers, students, and patients, looking beyond familiar territory, searching for new possibilities for methods mastered, taught, and successfully practised. For our mutual benefit, John Cross has laid down for us a detailed path for us to follow to experience the remarkable and fascinating power of human touch and the 'circuitry of the body' Until recently, interactions of this kind have been difficult for those with conventional medical and biomedical training to comprehend, in spite of extensive documentation of mechanisms and clinical efficacy. Clearing the way to broader recognition are the profound clinical benefits and growing public acceptance of acupressure, acupuncture, and related methods. 'A picture is worth a thousand words,' and a satisfied patient is worth dozens of double-blind, placebo-controlled, statistical studies.

Acupressure by John Cross is a detailed and brilliantly illustrated handbook for those who wish to enhance their therapeutic effectiveness. It is an important contribution to the exciting changes that are sweeping through health care systems world-wide.

James L Oschman, PhD
Author of *Energy Medicine: The Scientific Basis*
Harcourt Brace, 2000

Introduction

This book is written with the earnest desire that the subjects covered and the treatments described will, in time, become part of the standard physical therapy as taught today. The author has for many years taught these techniques and methods to chartered physiotherapists and other medical professionals, and has received enough feedback to warrant putting the material into print. There has for some time been a number of books on the subject of acupressure and touch therapy that have been aimed at the lay public and interested professionals. This book is aimed solely at the practising physical therapist, and gives a *total treatment* approach, thus giving the therapist a real alternative to the more orthodox methods usually employed in physiotherapy.

The most important thing to realize when one starts to learn acupressure is that it is *different*. This probably sounds a silly thing to say – 'of course it is different', you are saying, 'otherwise we would all be taught it as standard in our colleges and schools'. What is meant by being *different* is that one is dealing with a different concept, different philosophy and different techniques to those of ordinary massage. When I have a student therapist working with me and they see me just gently holding two points on the patient's body, seemingly at random, they usually ask the obvious questions, 'Why are you doing that?' and 'Surely that isn't enough to achieve anything?'. I find that the most simple questions are often the most difficult to answer. My 25 years experience of using Chinese massage has given me more insight and intuition, and has enabled me to perform treatments without going into the whys and wherefores. This book will explain all the whys and wherefores in a logical way so that students and experienced therapists alike will be able to understand more of how the body really works and, by having that knowledge, can eventually become more intuitive. The secret is to accept the underlying philosophy and stand by it; it will be your friend. We become unstuck when we fall between two stools and attempt to practise using many philosophies and theories – it cannot be done!

I believe that there is a time for everything. Although I could have written this book 10 years ago, it would not have been accepted either by the publisher or by the therapist. We have moved on from the days when I was told not to place my physiotherapy qualifications alongside my acupuncture letters on my headed note paper; we are living in a more enlightened time, where the use of acupuncture, herbal medicine, homeopathy, osteopathy etc. are commonplace, even in the most stringently orthodox circles. By writing about acupressure and by discussing the use of massage, we are surely going back to the roots of our noble profession. I have stated literally hundreds of times from the lectern that we should be able to throw away *all* our electrical machines and get back to using our hands as our main treatment modality. With our hands we get feel and feedback; we don't get that with machines. God gave us hands before He gave us a plug on the wall – USE THEM!!

1

History of acupressure

Acupressure has been used in healing for over 5000 years, and has many guises, methods and theories. It is important to appreciate all the traditional and modern aspects of this healing art in order that therapists can understand and disseminate all the theories presented and be able to choose to which type they are best suited. Chartered physiotherapists, osteopaths and chiropractors are well equipped to learn and practise the methods shown, as they already have had a 'hands on' training and understand the anatomical and physiological complexities of the human body. Whatever the type of acupressure that is practised, it is essentially a type of healing that deals with *touch* and *feel*. Many a sceptical physiotherapist has started a course in acupressure with an ice-like approach to learning a new modality, only to be totally converted within a few hours.

The knowledge that massage and touch improves a person's general health and eases pain dates from prehistoric times. The earliest text describing touch as a healing modality is the *Huang Ti Nei Ching* (*Yellow Emperor's Manual of Corporeal Medicine*). This gives, together with needle acupuncture and the use of diet, herbs and moxa, a detailed account of our relationship with the elements, time, seasons and weather systems, as well as of internal imbalances that have an effect on our general wellbeing. It is believed that acupressure originated in India and later spread to China, Egypt and Asia by Buddhist monks. It was also quaintly thought that warriors returning from war exhibiting spear or arrow wounds would be slowly healed of other discomfort and disease as their wounds healed, the site of the wound bearing no relationship to the diseased organ or body part that improved.

Over the years and decades, points have been mapped out on the body that have an influence on a certain internal organ if they are stimulated. These points are called *acupoints* or *tsubo*. Points on the body that possessed a similar organ affinity were 'joined together' by a series of invisible channels or networks called *meridians*, and each of the meridians was given the name of the organ that it influenced. There are 14 named meridians, of which 12 are associated with organs that we understand in orthodox medicine and two are unilateral. There are an additional six meridians that are mixes and composites of the others, making 20 meridians in all (18 bilateral and two unilateral). Acupoints are located in particular places on the skin and are usually quite easy to find and detect in that they lie either proximal or distal to certain bony prominences or in hollows made naturally by muscular or tendinous intersections. There are only a few situated in 'obscure' places. What has fascinated me since the time I started to learn this art is the way in which doctors could *know* when they were affecting a particular point. There must have been, originally, some kind of insight or intuition on their part. Knowledge was then passed down from teacher to students and offspring.

Traditional Chinese medicine

As today, in the times that traditional Chinese medicine was in its infancy patients were all shapes and sizes – fat or thin, tall or short. Where was the yardstick to provide accurate measurement, since it could not be based on standard units or distance from one point to another using imperial measure? Under the Han Dynasty (202 BCE–220 CE) a solution was found by taking a relative physical measurement, the *cun* (*tchun*) or *pouce*, as the unit of measurement. The patient's own body shape was used, and 1 cun was the width of the patient's thumb at its widest part, which is also equal to the distance between the extent of the skin crease at the distal two joints of the middle finger. Figure 1.1 shows the measurements of the body in terms of cun.

This unit of measurement is still used today by student practitioners although, with experience, the location of the points will become automatic. Having said that, generally when points need treatment they are painful (see Chapter 4).

Vital force

The Chinese have practised acupressure both on themselves and on others for over 5000 years as a way of maintaining health – not necessarily to ease symptoms or to cure. They believe that in the meridians there flows an invisible life force energy called *Ch'i*. It is the manipulation of Ch'i at the acupoints by stimulation or touch that creates a balance of energy where there was previously an imbalance. In traditional terms, disease = dis-ease = imbalance of energy, and the restoration of balance = health. The correlation that is often used with energy flow and the meridians is to imagine the meridian system to be like a canal or waterway system, and the acupoints as the lock gates along the canal. When the point is stimulated the lock gate is opened and the water flows through, energy once more flowing freely through the system. This is a terribly basic, almost naïve, illustration, but in practice it seems to work. In acupressure, the experienced therapist can actually *feel* the flow of energy.

It is said that Ch'i energy is an all-pervading and powerful force that exists in every cell in the body. The flow of Ch'i can best be manipulated at the acupoints, in particular those points between the

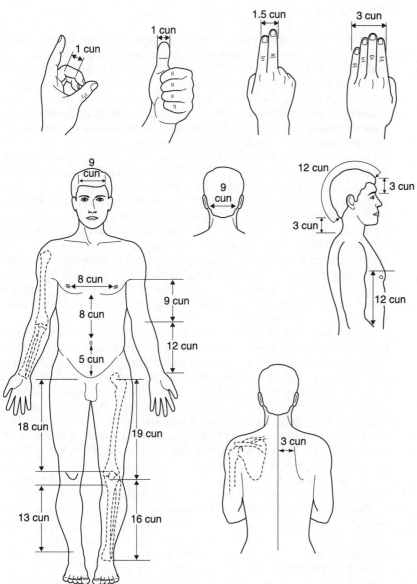

Figure 1.1 The Chinese inch: cun or pouce measurements.

elbow and the fingers and those between the knee and the toes. These are called *command* points. In each meridian there are one or two *great* or influential points that are used more than any other, as experience has shown that they are more effective than others. Exactly what Ch'i is has been argued about for centuries, but it is, of course, just one interpretation of *vital* or *life force*. Views on this and other 'energies' will be dealt with later in this chapter and in Chapter 6.

From the viewpoint of traditional Chinese medicine philosophy, there are four components that must be considered in order to increase the knowledge and awareness of this wonderful form of healing. These are Yin and Yang, the time clock, the law of five elements, and the traditional eight approaches to disease and healing.

Yin and Yang

These two words (pronounced 'inn' and 'arng') are the two bi-polars of Ch'i, and are opposite and yet complementary to each other. Yin and Yang philosophy is deeply embedded in traditional medicines of many kinds, not just Chinese. They form the backbone of thought in traditional Indian, Japanese, Huna and tribal medicines. A deep knowledge of the bi-polar forces of Yin and Yang can explain many things about the cosmos itself, as well as about the human body, but for the purposes of this book we will stick to the salient points needed for our understanding of the concept in the treatment of physical illness. Yang covers the acute side of disease, whereas Yin covers the chronic. Table 1.1 gives a few Yang and Yin equivalents.

Figure 1.2 shows the symbol known as the *pakua* or the Chinese monad. This indicates wholeness which, according to the Chinese, is simply Ch'i. The shaded area is Yin and the light area is Yang. Note that the division is not a straight line but a curved one – nothing in nature or the human frame is straight; nothing is black and white but all is various shades of grey. Note also that there is a little Yin in the Yang, and a little Yang in the Yin. Put in therapy terms, one can never have a wholly Yin or Yang condition. Total Yin is, of course, death of the physical body.

As nothing in medicine is totally Yin or Yang, for the remainder of the book we will discuss conditions as being predominantly Yin or Yang, meaning that they are chronic or acute. Generally speaking, where there is a Yang condition there is pain, inflammation, heat and redness, and this condition needs to be *sedated* (in order to balance the energy). Where there is a Yin condition there is also pain, but it is sluggish, stiff, chronic, oedematous etc., and this needs to be *stimulated*. There is a golden rule of thumb in most therapies that the acute needs to be addressed first before the chronic nature of the dis-ease can be unravelled. This is certainly true in acupressure. The same point can be used to stimulate or sedate, depending on the way it is treated, hence giving a different sensation and result.

The internal organs can also be placed in a Yin/Yang context as follows:

Small intestine	Heart
Large intestine	Lung
Bladder	Kidney
Gall bladder	Liver
Stomach	Spleen
Triple heater	Pericardium
Governor	Conception

These have been placed in no particular order, but it is important they are memorized as Yin/Yang couples. The latter two pairs will be explained later. Note that the Yang organs are hollow, peristaltic and not vital to life, whereas the Yin organs are solid organs that are essential to life. I appreciate that one can do without the spleen and one kidney, but these organs control far more than Western medicine appreciates. The spleen, for instance, is said to be the home of the immune system, and has important uses in gynaecological conditions.

Table 1.1 Yin and Yang equivalents

Yang	*Yin*
Summer	Winter
Heat	Cold
Male	Female
Light	Dark
Acute	Chronic
Spastic	Flaccid
Mobility	Stiffness
Inflammation	Oedema
Hypertension	Hypotension
Hollow organs	Vital organs

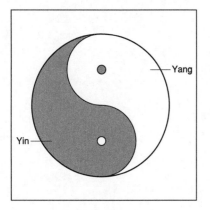

Figure 1.2 The Chinese monad.

The Chinese time clock

Ch'i energy flows in the meridians in a precise and logical manner during the 24-hour cycle. There is always energy in each of the organs, but for 2 hours in each 24 hours there is more energy in a particular organ than in any other. For example, the heart energy peaks at 1100 and is at its least at 2300 hrs. Kidney energy peaks at 1700 and is at its least at 0500 hrs. This information is very useful for the therapist, both in knowing the hour of the day that one should treat a particular condition and for the knowledge that it may be normal for a particular organ or system to exhibit certain symptoms at particular times of the day and not others. It would be abnormal, for instance, for the stomach to have excess energy in the evening, and if it does this shows signs of imbalance.

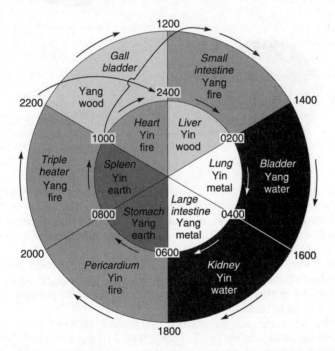

Figure 1.3 The Chinese time clock.

The Chinese clock (Figure 1.3) gives the therapist the ideal time to treat a certain condition – for example, 1400–1800 hrs for osteoarthritis (bladder and kidney meridian association) and 1000–1400 hrs is the ideal time to treat chronic muscular imbalance (gall bladder and liver association). Knowledge of this clock is also useful in the treatment of jet lag, when the body's clock is out of phase with the local time.

The law of five elements (transformations)

As with Yin and Yang, there have been large, complex books written on this Law alone, so here it is simplified, mentioning only those aspects that the therapist needs to know.

Each organ is placed in one of five 'elements', the Yang organs being on the outside and the Yin on the inside, with the Yin/Yang

Figure 1.4 The law of the five elements.

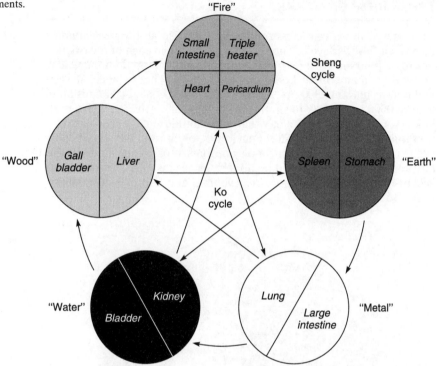

couple opposite each other (Figure 1.4). The *Sheng* or engendering cycle is said to be the creative cycle, and the *Ko* cycle is said to be the controlling cycle. The five elements are not chemical elements, but rather five aspects of the world, nature and the human frame that represent the rhythms of life.

In the Sheng cycle, fire produces ashes (earth); earth (as ore) produces metal; metal produces water through hydrolysis; water produces wood in the sense that water makes plant life possible; wood makes fire as in fuel.

In the Ko cycle, fire subjugates metal as in melting; metal subjugates wood as in cutting or chopping; wood subjugates earth by penetrating it with roots; earth subjugates water by absorbing it or providing a dam or obstruction; water subjugates fire by extinguishing it.

Table 1.2 represents a fraction of the many and various aspects of this law and shows what can be placed into each element.

Examples of clinical importance

1. Patients can sometimes be archetyped according to which system and part of the body is affected. Knowing this, the therapist can treat the relevant meridian and acupoints.
2. As will be revealed in a later chapter, Ch'i energy can be transferred from element to element, thus providing a balance of energies within the body.
3. By taking a correct case history the therapist will be able to ascertain how condition has followed condition, seemingly at random but actually always in a logical plan according to the Ko cycle.

Table 1.2 The law of five elements

	Fire	*Earth*	*Metal*	*Water*	*Wood*
Direction	South	–	West	North	East
Colour	Red	Yellow	White	Black	Green
System	Circulation	Connective tissue	Skin	Bones	Muscles
Sense	Speech	Taste	Smell	Hearing	Sight
Face	Mouth	Tongue	Nose	Ears	Eyes
Emotion	Excess joy	Depression	Grief	Fear	Anger
Season	Summer	Late summer	Autumn (fall)	Winter	Spring
Taste	Bitter	Sweet	Pungent	Salt	Sour
Weather	Heat	Humidity	Dryness	Cold	Wind

With any form of natural healing, of which acupressure is one, patients will heal themselves in a 'reverse-Ko' manner, and disease is slowly eradicated.

4. Take, for example someone who has chronic osteoarthritis of the knees. If, on questioning, it is found that the problem is worse in cold (winter) and the person possibly has hearing difficulties or itchy ears and/or a taste for salty things, one can deduce that he or she is very much a Water person and needs to have the kidney and bladder meridians strengthened as well as the 'mother' of Water, namely Metal, stimulated. This means that acupressure treatment needs to be centred on the source points of the relevant meridians, plus the Water point of the lung/large intestine meridians. This is performed prior to treatment on the knees. It is useless to give therapy symptomatically if the general Ch'i energy has not been addressed – we may just as well give patients allopathic medicine to treat the symptoms!

The eight approaches

The traditional Chinese doctor (or barefoot doctor, as they were known) makes a thorough and comprehensive examination of the patient and takes a case history, approaching the patient gently and considerately. The doctor first observes and listens to the patient, then touches and palpates the body, reads the pulses, looks at the tongue, looks at the eyes and palpates the abdomen. The findings of the clinical examination are put under the eight key-symptoms or approaches of Chinese medicine: Deep and Superficial; Cold and Heat; Emptiness and Fullness; and finally Yin and Yang. These differentiations enable the doctor to ascertain the energetic imbalance and determine the severity of the ailment. Emptiness indicates an energy deficiency and includes such symptoms as lack of appetite, night sweats and lassitude. Fullness indicates an acute disorder and includes symptoms such as excess phlegm, flatulence and constipation. If the patient does not feel thirsty or prefers hot drinks there is a Cold disorder, whereas thirst for cold drinks, dry lips, red eyes and general restlessness are symptoms of Heat. Pains in the peripheral joints are called Superficial, and pains in the chest and abdomen are called Deep. Yin and Yang are the basic principles for the functioning of the whole organism and also describe the others; hence Yang can cover Superficial, Heat and Fullness, and Yin can cover Cold, Deep and Emptiness. Quite often, as in Western medicine, the object of the treatment is to convert a chronic condition into an acute one in order to make it easier to treat; thus we attempt to turn Cold into Heat, Deep into Superficial, Emptiness into Fullness and Yin into Yang.

Traditional Japanese medicine

There are many facets of traditional Japanese thought, and much of it is similar to traditional Chinese philosophy. Many of the individual theories have combined to give us today the massage form known as *shiatsu*. The vital force in Japanese is called Ki (pronounced kee) and comes from the word *tanki*, which means 'heaven energy'. Like the Chinese counterpart of Ch'i, it is an all-embracing and all-pervading energy system and has a deeply rooted philosophy that is not only concerned with medicine but with the weather, seasons and life itself. The Japanese equivalent of Yang is Jitsu, and of Yin is Kyo. The meridians are the same, except that the numbering on them is slightly different and more emphasis is made in healing of the Jitsu channels.

Shiatsu is a Japanese word made up of two written characters meaning finger (*shi*) and pressure (*atsu*). The acupuncture points used in shiatsu are called *tsubo*, and treatment consists of pressure on these and broad areas using the fingers, thumbs, elbows and feet. Whereas the traditional form of massage in general terms in China is called *anmo*, in Japan it is called *anma*. Anma became a healing art that was associated with blind people and even now, of course, people with impaired vision quite often make excellent 'hands-on' therapists. Shiatsu therapy started to be associated with folklore when orthodox medicine began to take over as the main medical armamentum, but since the Second World War these ancient forms of healing have started to re-emerge.

It is ironic that shiatsu is now most popular in the Western world, especially in Britain and the USA, and that it has recently taken somewhat of a dive in popularity in Japan, where it has been replaced by more subtle forms of healing. Shiatsu tends to be quite aggressive but it is excellent in the treatment of many mechanical and physical complaints (mention is made of some shiatsu methods in later chapters), although it is not for the fainthearted either to practise or to be practised upon. Please do not get the impression that all shiatsu uses aggressive or violent massage – there is a form that is called Zen-shiatsu that is very passive. Shiatsu also adopts the holistic principles of the treatment of body–mind–spirit and accepts all the naturopathic laws.

Traditional Indian (esoteric) touch therapy

Up until recently, use of the *chakras* and the other higher centres of energy has been reserved for the traditional Eastern medicines and religions and in the practice of yoga and meditation. Information from various ancient texts of Indian yogic literature give mention to these special force centres or chakras that exist on the surface of the body, having many internal relationships and associations (including nerve plexii and endocrine glands) and yet having a more subtle (or more powerful) association with our bodies and aura. The word *chakra* means 'wheel' in Sanskrit, and chakras are considered to be whirling vortices of energy that exist as acupuncture points on the body's surface and balloon outwards into our etheric and astral bodies in the shape of an expanding cornet. Each chakra has particular anatomical landmarks, and each is represented by a different vibrational rate, colour, endocrine gland, nerve plexus and set of symptoms (should any imbalance occur). There are seven major chakras that have dorsal and ventral aspects, together with 21 minor chakras that are all aspected by an acupoint, each being a reflected point of a major chakra and having its own characteristics in healing. It has been the author's onerous but pleasant task over the past 15 years to attempt to explain the chakra energy system in western orthodox terms. The role of chakras in clinical acupressure when treating musculo-skeletal conditions is quite significant, and will be mentioned later in the book.

Philosophers and vital force

It would be helpful now to mention a little more about what the Chinese call Ch'i, the Japanese call Ki and the Indians call Prana – in other words, vital or life force – and how different great philosophers down the ages have interpreted it.

Pythagorus (b. 590 BCE) was a philosopher, mathematician and astronomer. He was also a physician – the 'noblest of all'. He called this life energy *pneuma*, and said that it came from a central fire in the universe and provided man with his vitality and immortal soul.

Hippocrates (b. 460 BCE), the father of holistic medicine, called the energy *medicatrix naturae*. He said that disease is the body's attempt to re-establish harmony, that illness is sometimes beneficial and that we should never just meddle with the symptoms. (Some 2000 years later, we still haven't got our act together regarding holism).

Paracelsus (b. 1493 CE) was one of the most brilliant physicians that the world has ever seen. He believed in a healing energy that radiated within and around man like a luminous sphere, which he called *archaeus*. He said that it operated at a distance and was able to both cause and cure disease. He was the founder of magnetic healing.

Franz Anton Mesmer (1733–1815) was convinced, like Paracelsus, that humans were influenced by a force of subtle energy in the universe (cosmos) that could be harnessed for healing purposes. Mesmer called this energy simply *animal magnetism*, and spent most of his life working with magnets, magnetic force and healing. After a while he realized that he did not need magnets in order to heal, and simply laid hands on his patients in order to cure, much to the annoyance of the medical fraternity. By the time he was in his thirties he was recognized as a great healer, not only with his hands but also by the power of suggestion and thought. He 'invented' hypnotism as we know it today, but for years it was called *mesmerism*. This system was later copied by Mary Baker Eddy to become the foundation (with a few variations) of Christian Science.

Baron Karl Von Reichenberg (b. 1788) was a German born scientist who shocked the world of orthodox medical science with his views on healing energy. He called it *Od* or *Odic force* (from the Norse God Odin, meaning great power). He was convinced that this force permeated all nature, and he spent 30 years of his life trying to prove it. He was convinced that Od was the link between science and the supernatural, but like most philosophers and deep thinkers was ahead of his time. He was ridiculed as a charlatan, and spent many lonely years in exile.

William Reich (1902–1957) was a psychiatrist and natural scientist. He was convinced that he had found the secret of all creation in what he called *orgone* energy, a mass-free primordial power that operated throughout the universe as the basic life force. He described this energy as being present in all living things as well as the atmosphere and the earth, and said that proper flow of this energy force throughout the body was essential to health. He believed that it was related to variations in the earth's magnetism. He also believed the energy to be intelligent and it was, he conjected, the scientific reality of what most people consider to be God or Allah.

In the last few decades there have been very many great people of science, art, philosophy and medicine who have all engaged themselves in the study of life force. These include de la Warr and Drown (the doyens of radionics), Edgar Cayce, who was probably the most gifted natural healer of all time, Rudolf Steiner, Sigmund Freud, Carl Jung, Mary Baker Eddy, Leadbeater, David Tansley, Malcolm Rae and many others too numerous to mention. Each has dealt with life force in a different way and given it different connotations that range from the spiritual and religious to the psychotic and physical. In order to understand what acupressure really is, it is important to mention two great men of history, D. D. Palmer and Andrew Taylor Still, who each made his life's work the study of body therapeutics and hands-on healing and gave the world of medicine and physical therapy something new. Each has explained his different type of physical medicine in a new and exciting way, and both have opened up new frontiers in physical medicine.

D. D. Palmer is generally credited as having founded the manipulative art of chiropractic. Many people believe that he 'invented' it on 18 September 1895 in Davenport, Iowa, when he adjusted the third cervical vertebra of a deaf janitor called Harvey Lillard and restored his hearing as a result. Palmer insisted that there was a vital force or energy called *innate*. The innate was the power that kept the autonomic system functioning and expressed itself through the nervous system. Palmer emphasized that chiropractic does not cure; the adjustment relieves and removes the cause, then the life force (innate) transmits impulses without hindrances and effects a cure. Palmer's original ideas have either been accepted without question by other chiropractors (and indeed other disciplines of manipulation) or rejected out-of-hand as being too esoteric. The scientific branch of chiropractic feels that the health and wellbeing, as well as symptomatic pain relief, that one has after a chiropractic adjustment is due to the removal of various soft tissue blockages which, in turn, stimulates the flow of blood, lymph and nerve impulses. The author has found with experience that most disciplines comprise two schools of thought; those that follow the originator's ideas and others who attempt to quantify them scientifically. Such is true of many forms of physical therapy – homoeopathy, acupuncture etc. But let us return to physical medicine.

Andrew Taylor Still was the founder of osteopathy, and was born in 1828 in Virginia, the son of a Methodist minister. He went to medical school and then into the army, where he rose to the rank of major and became an army surgeon. He studied the human body, its structure and function in detail, and became convinced that only through the understanding of the vital connection between structure and function could an answer be found to disease and imbalances that occurred in the body. In 1864 an epidemic of meningitis struck the Missouri frontier and thousands died, including his three children. This desperate state made him study even harder to try and correlate a link between germ disease and the human frame. He came to the belief that a person should be treated as a whole; that a person cannot get sick in one area of the body without involvement of other parts or organs. He developed the art of manipulative therapy based on his detailed knowledge of human anatomy, physiology and the newly found inter-relationship between the body and its function. He found that by careful palpation of a patient's soft tissues he could ascertain organic imbalance, and that by gentle vertebral and soft tissue manipulation he was able to achieve startling results. He died in 1917 at the age of 89 years and left a legacy of over 10 000 osteopathic practitioners in the USA and Europe. Andrew Taylor Still will always be remembered for the simple and yet far-reaching statement: Structure governs function.

Of course there are many others who have founded and pioneered their own particular brands of physical medicine, but space does not allow mention of them in depth. Briefly, though, they include: W. G. Sutherland (founder of cranial osteopathy); George Goodheart (founder of applied kinesiology); John Upledger (founder of the modern concepts of cranio-sacral therapy); Tom Bowen (Bowen therapy); Fritz Smith (zero balancing); and Eunice Ingham (reflex zone therapy). Many others have also taken the traditional and modern aspects of hands-on therapies into new bounds. To them all, we owe a debt of gratitude.

2

Meridians and acupoints

The various aspects of Ch'i and how vital force can be interpreted are now discussed. This is mostly by the meridians, acupoints, zones and the scores of reflexes. People tend to get confused with these various approaches, but they needn't if they accept the philosophies at face value and don't try scientifically to analyse them too much. This chapter deals with meridians and acupoints.

Meridians

Mention has been made already that there are 12 bilateral meridians or energy channels, and that each one is related to and associated with an internal organ. There are also two unilateral meridians and six others that are composites of the main ones. These latter eight are known

Table 2.1 The 12 bilateral meridians and their relationships

'Peak' time	Meridian	Yin/Yang	Element	Direction of energy flow
0300	Lung	Yin	Metal	Chest to hand
0500	Large intestine	Yang	Metal	Hand to face (nose)
0700	Stomach	Yang	Earth	Face to foot
0900	Spleen	Yin	Earth	Foot to chest
1100	Heart	Yin	Fire	Chest to hand
1300	Small intestine	Yang	Fire	Hand to face (ear)
1500	Bladder	Yang	Water	Face to foot
1700	Kidney	Yin	Water	Foot to chest
1900	Pericardium	Yin	Fire	Chest to hand
2100	Triple heater	Yang	Fire	Hand to face (eye)
2300	Gall bladder	Yang	Wood	Face to foot
0100	Liver	Yin	Wood	Foot to chest

Table 2.2   Important points on the meridians

Meridian	Symbol	From	To	No. of points	Source	Accumu-lation	Great	Type
Stomach	St	Eye	2nd toe	45	42	41	36	Yang
Spleen	Sp	Great toe	6th intercostal space	21	3	2	6	Yin
Heart	Ht	Axilla	Little finger	9	7	9	7	Yin
Small intestine	Si	Little finger	Ear	19	4	3	3	Yang
Bladder	Bl	Eye	Little toe	67	64	67	62	Yang
Kidney	Ki	Sole of foot	Clavicle	27	3	7	6	Yin
Pericardium	P	Chest	Middle finger	9	7	9	6	Yin
Triple heater	TH	Ring finger	Ear	23	4	3	5	Yang
Gall bladder	GB	Eye	4th toe	44	40	43	42	Yang
Liver	Li	Great toe	Chest	14	3	8	3	Yin
Lung	Lu	Chest	Thumb	11	9	9	7	Yin
Large intestine	LI	Index finger	Nose	21	4	11	4	Yang

as the eight extraordinary meridians, but only the unilateral ones of the *governor* and *conception* need concern us. Although the others are more than useful when using acupuncture they tend not to be very effective or useful in acupressure, apart from the knowledge of their key points, which is important. Mention has been made of the Chinese time clock, and it would be useful here to place the meridians in the 'time clock' order. Each meridian has its 'peak' of energy over a 24-hour period, is either Yin or Yang, is associated with a particular element and has a direction of energy flow (Table 2.1).

Looking at Table 2.1, the reader can see that energy flows in a logical sequence from organ/meridian to organ/meridian. For example, with the arms outstretched above the head, Yin energy flows upwards and Yang energy flows downwards. This knowledge is very important, as the actual direction of energy flow will make all the difference in the several techniques of acupressure.

- There are three Yang–arm meridians: small intestine, large intestine and triple heater
- There are three Yin–arm meridians: heart, pericardium and lung
- There are three Yang–leg meridians: bladder, stomach and gall bladder
- There are three Yin–leg meridians: kidney, spleen and liver.

Yang meridians tend to lie on the posterior and lateral aspects of the limbs, whereas Yin meridians lie on the anterior and medial aspects. In a way it seems that the Yin meridians are protected and the Yang ones are open – thus mimicking the organs themselves.

The most influential acupressure points in the meridian system of energy are the command points, which are the points that lie between the elbow and fingers and between the knee and toes. Each meridian at the end of the limbs has some very important points: the *tsing* or nail point, the source point, the accumulation point and the great point. Occasionally these overlap, but not often.

The tsing point, being at the start of the meridian, varies in importance with the meridian. It is sometimes called the nail point, as it is

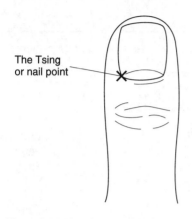

Figure 2.1   The tsing or nail point.

The Tsing
or nail point

always situated at the side of the nail. These are always painful points and care must be taken when treating them (Figure 2.1).

The source point is that point on the meridian that most easily affects the actual organ associated with the meridian.

The accumulation point is that point where energy can be transferred from one meridian to another, thus creating a balance of energy.

The great point is the most important point on the meridian in that it can serve more than one function. If readers wish just to memorize the great points, then they will not go far wrong in their knowledge and practice of meridian acupressure.

Figure 2.2 shows the meridians.

So what is a meridian? And what is an acupoint? These are questions that have baffled scientists for many years. We seem very close now to having a scientific rationale for the existence of acupoints, but the existence of meridians remains a scientifically unknown commodity. As Western acupuncture (and hence scientific acupuncture) seems to be obsessed with only the analgesic effects of acupuncture and acupressure, almost to the detriment of every other factor, research trials were set up along the lines of trying to prove the efficacy of analgesic acupuncture. Research has been performed *ad nauseum* throughout the world comparing the anaesthetic effects of non-acupuncture points (sham acupuncture) with recognized acupoints. It has been clearly demonstrated that a significant analgesic effect occurs using true acupuncture points compared with little effect using sham acupuncture (Chapman *et al.*, 1977). The results in alleviating chronic pain are not so convincing, but various studies have shown a 45–50 per cent reduction in pain. The placebo effect in these results cannot be ruled out; indeed, there are bound to be placebo effects during any double-blind trials. Shrenberger (1977) attempted to show the existence of meridians in cadavers by using electro-analysis. It is amazing to think that some people actually believed this, when after all we are supposed to be dealing with a life force and not a death force!! Zong-Xiang (1981) suggested that a meridian channel is a transmission pathway for low resistance points on that line. Becker (1976) seems to support this, as does Tiberiu (1981). Lazorthes (1990) stated that meridians can be made visible with staining. The results of his work showed that the visible pathways were in fact vascular drainage channels. Later on Vernejoul (1992) conducted further research involving injections of radiotracers at acupoints and suggested that meridians are deeper pathways than the traditional concept and that channels are not related to either vascular drainage or lymphatic channels. He also stated that the migration speed along the channel differs in velocity and the movement is bidirectional, and thus suggests a neurochemical mechanism of information. So far, though, the scientific evidence for the existence of meridians is relatively weak. The research that has taken place to prove the existence of acupoints is, however, much more substantial. Literally thousands of trials and experiments have concluded that acupoints do exist. They seem to be points on the body's skin that show a lower electrical resistance compared to the surrounding tissues. It seems, therefore, that we are willing to accept that these points (acupoints, tsubo, reflex and trigger) exist, but that meridians (as laid down in classical acupuncture charts) do not. Does this matter to the effectiveness of acupres-

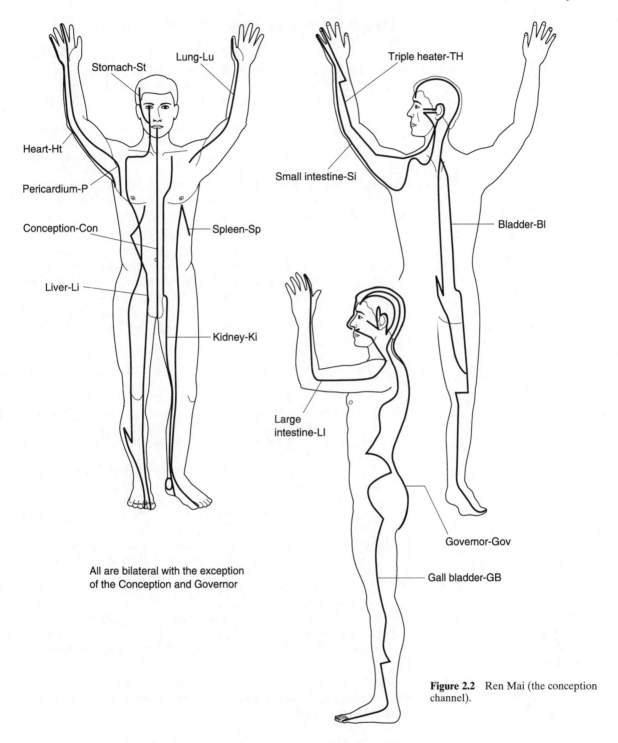

Stomach-St

Lung-Lu

Heart-Ht

Pericardium-P

Conception-Con

Spleen-Sp

Liver-Li

Kidney-Ki

Triple heater-TH

Small intestine-Si

Bladder-Bl

Large intestine-LI

Governor-Gov

Gall bladder-GB

All are bilateral with the exception of the Conception and Governor

Figure 2.2 Ren Mai (the conception channel).

sure and to the treatment of medical and physical conditions? Of course not!! Science can only prove that which is scientifically provable, and the author would respectfully suggest that the existence of Ch'i cannot be proved with scientific gadgetry.

Western physiology versus traditional Chinese physiology

So far there have been three main theories (or sets of theories) as to how acupuncture and acupressure work using Western physiological concepts; the thalamus theory, the 'gate' theory of pain and the Deqi theory.

The thalamus theory

Walter Thompson, in the first Korth lecture (Thompson, 1973) and later in his book entitled *Personalised Diagnosis* (published privately), states that 'it is the THALAMUS that is the centre of acupuncture reasoning and it is there that our future research should be channelled'. He concludes that:

1. Each cell in the brain is responsible for a particular duty and that, in order to be able to work in close proximity without interference with the adjacent cells, its plasma membrane has a special type of insulating quality, selecting and accepting only messages of micro-wavelength to which its own cell is tuned.
2. The transmission of these messages of micro-frequency is initiated by chemo-electrical conversion in the skin membranes etc. by all five senses.
3. The position or location of the point of initiation of the message relative to the brain plays some part in determining the individual wavelength.
4. The over-excitation of any of these initiating forces by higher frequencies outside the normal tuned reception wavelength has the effect of jamming the receiving cell, probably at the synapse, and stopping it from performing its normal duty in its target area; hence anaesthesia.
5. Ch'i energy in the pathways of acupuncture meridians from pore to brain may be chemo-electrical or chemical by the merging of chemicals (especially DNA) both along the line and at the initiating pore, all finally being converted from blood and other fluids in the midbrain.
6. From the brain and the central nervous system, acupuncture messages pass via the thalamus to operate as normal endocrine functions and transmission methods and achieve the target function.
7. The acupoints are probably the answer to the many little-understood functions of the body and brain, such as extrasensory perception, telepathy and psychic phenomena (particularly in animals), radiation to and from the body, aura etc., besides the acceptance of light/colour (photosynthesis) frequencies, and therefore may be our 'sixth sense'.

There is quite an overflow of holistic thought in Walter Thompson's work, and he is to be highly commended for his groundbreaking thesis and theories.

The 'gate' theory of pain

Another thought on the Western physiological theories of acupuncture and acupressure concerns the 'gate' theory of pain. Dr George Lewith, in his book *Modern Chinese Acupuncture*, writes:

All pain input enters the spinal cord via the substantia gelatinosa, pain impulses travelling along the small nerve fibres closing the gate to the pain at the caudal level, within the substantia gelatinosa. If pain is not transmitted to the brain, no pain is perceived.

(Lewith and Lewith, 1994)

Melzack (1977) has suggested that acupressure stimulates large myelinated nerve fibres, thereby closing the gate to pain. But, as Dr Lewith points out, there are a large number of problems with the 'gate' theory, particularly as it is used to explain the mechanism of acupuncture/pressure, and because there is much more to acupressure than its analgesic effect, there must be other plausible explanations.

The Deqi theory

In her excellent book *Acupuncture in Clinical Practice*, Nadia Ellis (1994) has the following to add:

> To get an analgesic effect it is important to achieve Deqi. This is a heavy sensation that is felt around the point when needling (this happens in sustained acupressure too) within the acupoint. If a subcutaneous injection of procaine is given prior to inserting the needle, the deqi is not affected; however, if a similar injection is given deep into the muscle in the acupoint area there is a inhibition of deqi (Chang and Chang, 1983). It can logically be concluded in the light of these findings that the main components for deqi are carried by the small myelinated afferents from the muscle. In the case of superficial acupoints not sited in muscles, the response is through the peripheral nerves so that the A-delta fibres are stimulated. Impulses are sent to the spinal cord and are transmitted up the antero-lateral tract to activate three centres:
>
> 1. Spinal cord at the lateral horn where enkephalin and dymorphin block messages at low frequency and other transmitters, not fully identified, at high frequency. The anaelgesic effect of high frequency stimulation is short lived, lasting very little time after the stimulation stops.
> 2. Midbrain. This uses enkephalin to activate the raphe descending system, which inhibits the spinal cord pain transmission by the synergic effect of the monoamines, serotonin and norepinephrine.
> 3. Pituitary/hypothalamus. The pituitary is where B-endorphin is released into the circulation and the cerebrospinal fluid; thus completing the pain relieving process from a distance. The hypothalamus has connections with the midbrain and sends out long axons which, via B-endorphins activate the descending analgesia system.

These explanations are all fine when it comes to many forms of acupuncture and some forms of stimulating acupressure, but they fall short in explaining why the other types of acupressure work. They can never explain the fundamental life force that is within and without each and every one of us. It can be said that the work achieved with biochemistry, although it is excellent, falls short in explaining *how* it all works. We have positive results with every form and type of acupuncture and acupressure in hundreds of different medical conditions, and simple biochemistry cannot explain it all; it cannot explain the *root* of healing!

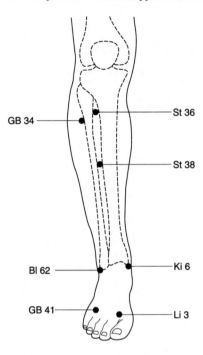

Figure 2.3 Anterior aspect of lower leg.

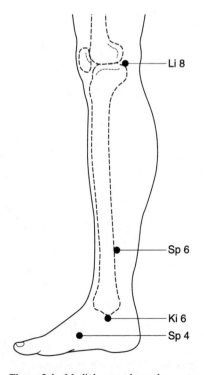

Figure 2.4 Medial aspect lower leg.

Great points

Great points are those points that have more energic 'quality' than other points. They normally have more than one function or action, and there is only one per meridian. There are, of course, many more than 12 important acupressure points, and these will be discussed later. The great points are as follows:

Stomach meridian	St 36	Spleen meridian	Sp 6
Heart meridian	Ht 7	Pericardium meridian	P 6
Small intestine meridian	Si 3	Three heater meridian	TH 5
Kidney meridian	Ki 6	Bladder meridian	Bl 62
Lung meridian	Lu 7	Large intestine meridian	LI 4
Liver meridian	Li 3	Gall bladder meridian	GB 41

The stomach meridian – St 36

St 36 lies one finger's breadth from the anterior crest of the tibia, between it and the fibula. (Figure 2.3).
Uses:

1. General tonification of energy of the body by stimulating massage.
2. Any upper gastro-intestinal tract imbalance, e.g. nausea, vomiting, gastralgia. To make someone vomit the contents of the stomach, heavy stimulation is needed. To calm down a gastralgia, light massage or gentle touch is needed.
3. Migraine, especially when pain settles over one eye and the cause can be attributed to the eating of a migraine 'trigger' food.
4. Infra-patellar knee pain.
5. Vagus nerve imbalance, i.e. vertigo or dizziness.
6. Upper palate toothache. Gentle pressure is needed here.

It is obvious to the reader that not all the attributes of St 36 are those of musculo-skeletal use; the object in describing the other uses is to give the reader a flavour of what else acupressure can be used for. The same is true of the remainder of the great points.

The spleen meridian – Sp 6

Sp 6 is situated 3 cun (Chinese inches) superior to the medial malleolus just posterior to the tibial border. (Figure 2.4).
Uses:

1. Restoration of energy in cases of general weakness.
2. Gastro-intestinal conditions.
3. Internal inflammations and ulcerations of the uterus and ovaries.
4. Intra-uterine bleeding and bleeding haemorrhoids.
5. Anaesthesia – general point.
6. Shin splints – local point.
7. Gravitational ulcer – parallel point.

Sp 6 is simply *the* great point in uterine conditions. Its anaesthetic qualities are best enhanced if used in conjunction with LI 4. It is very useful in period pain and also in permitting an easier childbirth. In conjunction with St 36 it is used in restoring vitality in cases of general weakness. Stimulating massage is needed for this.

The heart meridian – Ht 7

This point is situated on the ulnar side of the wrist on the posterior border of the pisiform bone (Figure 2.5).
Uses:

1. Nervous anxiety such as stage fright or examination nerves.
2. Sleeplessness due to anxiety or stress. Strong rhythmical massage is needed here, maybe combined with a little sheep counting!
3. Emotional trauma. One of the best uses of this point that is not mentioned in other texts but seems to work is that of emotional 'blockage' removal – as in bottling of emotions after a death in the family or similar emotional trauma. The heart meridian tends to 'soak up' this tension and can certainly be released by gentle yet firm manipulation of Ht 7 combined with LI 4.
4. Localized wrist pain such as carpal tunnel syndrome.
5. Axilla discomfort – distant point.

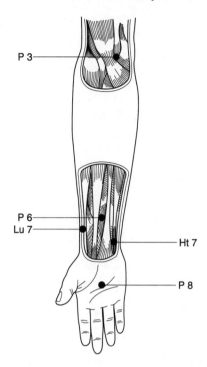

Figure 2.5 Anterior aspect of lower arm showing Ht 7 and P 6.

The pericardium meridian – P 6

This point is situated 2 cun proximal to the anterior wrist crease in the mid-line of the forearm (Figure 2.5).
Uses:

1. Insomnia, together with Ht 7.
2. Palpitation and angina pectoris pain, by itself or with LI 4.
3. Pain in the chest and costal region.
4. Hiccoughs.
5. General poor circulation and breakdown of blood patency.
6. Nausea, especially with travel sickness and early pregnancy.
7. It is one of the key points of the eight extraordinary meridians, with its couple being Sp 4.

The three heater meridian – TH 5

This point is situated 2 cun superior to the posterior wrist crease in the mid-line of the forearm (Figure 2.6). It directly opposes P 6 and a clever acupuncturist can actually lace a needle through P6 and pierce the skin on the opposite side of the forearm at TH 5. The author has seen this done at an acupuncture college, followed by much fainting of the viewing students! Needless to say this cannot be done in acupressure, and the two have to be treated individually.
Uses:

1. As the main point for 'bringing heat down' from the face and chest – it is excellent for hot flushes.

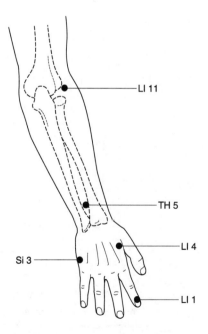

Figure 2.6 Posterior aspect of lower arm.

2. Paralysis of the sternocleidomastoid and upper fibres of the trapezius muscle (torticollis).
3. Deafness due to catarrh.
4. Fever.
5. Cold hands.
6. This point is also one of the key points of the eight extraordinary meridians, with GB as its couple. It is also the key point of the crown chakra based at Gov 20.

The small intestine meridian – Si 3

Si 3 is situated proximal to the fifth metacarpo-phalangeal joint on the ulnar border of the hand. (Figure 2.6).
    Uses:

1. Diarrhoea – stimulation.
2. Constipation – gentle massage.
3. Posterior shoulder pain, trigeminal neuralgia and elbow pain, either by itself or with other points.
4. Localized metacarpal pain.
5. It is one of the key points of the eight extraordinary meridians (governor channel), forming a couple with Bl 62. It is used in many spinal complaints because of this association.

The kidney meridian – Ki 6

This point is situated 1 cun below the tip of the medial malleolus. (Figure 2.3).
    Uses:

1. Treatment of the sexual organs, such as painful menstruation, scrotal pain and uterus prolapse.
2. Pain relief for pain on the antero-medial aspect of the torso, pubic area and groin, genital area and adductors.
3. Localized medial ankle pain.
4. It is one of the key points of the eight extraordinary meridians, with its couple being Lu 7.
5. It is one of the great 'energy' points, and as such can be used in such conditions as chronic fatigue syndrome as well as other conditions where tiredness plays a major part. It is also one of the major 'focal' or visualization points in certain types of Tai Chi or Qi Gong.

The bladder meridian – Bl 62

This point is situated half a cun directly inferior to the distal end of the lateral malleolus. (Figure 2.3).
    Uses:

1. Pain relief for such conditions as low back pain, sciatica, dorsal and cervical pain. It is one of the very great points in pain relief in these cases.
2. Localized lateral ankle pain.

3. It is one of the key points of the eight extraordinary meridians, with its couple being Si 3.
4. Lateral knee pain.

The lung meridian – Lu 7

This point is situated on the radial side of the forearm, 1.5 cun proximal to the transverse wrist crease. (Figure 2.5).
    Uses:

1. Obstructive airways diseases such as acute and chronic bronchitis, emphysema and asthma. Lu 7 is said to be the 'oxygen' point of the lung, and is useful in such cases.
2. Congestive sinusitis and catarrh.
3. It is the key point of the conception meridian (Ren Mai), with its couple being Ki 6.
4. Headaches of the 'brain-fag' type – used either by itself or in combination with LI 4 – also in facial pain and toothache.

The large intestine meridian (colon) – LI 4

LI 4 is situated on the highest point of the first interosseous muscle (adductor pollicis) when the thumb is adducted. (Figure 2.6).
    Uses:

1. Pain relief for the face, head, front and lateral aspect of shoulder and elbow.
2. Pain relief for the dorsum of the neck and occiput, also sinusitis and toothache of the lower jaw.
3. Constipation.
4. Skin conditions, especially acne of the face.
5. Localized tenosynovitis.
6. It is also used in combination with other points as follows:
        with Li 3 in calming
        with Lu 7 in clearing throat and chest congestion and pain
        with Si 2 or Si 3 in nosebleeds
        with Ht 7 in insomnia and nightmares.

This point is affectionately called 'the great eliminator', and is probably the most used point in acupuncture and acupressure simply because of its power and versatility. It is, however, contraindicated in pregnancy and during menstruation.

The gall bladder meridian – GB 41

GB 41 is situated in the depression distal to the junction of the fourth and fifth metatarsals. (Figure 2.3).
    Uses:

1. Hemi-cranial headaches, frontal headaches and shoulder pain.
2. Biliousness and colic.
3. Tinnitus – in combination with other points.

4.   Pain in the hip and along the ilio-tibial tract.
5.   Pain and conditions of the torso and mid-axillary line rib pain.
6.   It is a key point of one of the eight extraordinary meridians, with its couple being TH5.

The liver meridian – Li 3

Li 3 is situated at the proximal aspect between the first and second metatarsals. (Figure 2.3).
    Uses:

1.   Calming the nerves and easing restlessness and anxiety – with LI 4.
2.   Headaches, especially behind the eyes and those due to a hangover.
3.   Mastitis.
4.   Muscular tiredness and an 'all gone' sensation.
5.   Cramp – this is the specific point for cramp regardless of where it is in the body, but is particularly effective in calf cramp. Many a sleepless night has been saved with the knowledge of this point. Very gentle touch only is required, with *no* stimulation.

Specific points used in musculo-skeletal conditions

The following represents a comprehensive (but not exhaustive) list of the points that the therapist is most likely to use when treating musculo-skeletal conditions. Some have been previously mentioned in the great points section. Only general acting points will be mentioned in this section, as local acting points around joints will be mentioned in detail in the relevant chapter on the treatment of the individual joint conditions.

The lung meridian

Lu 1 – Zhongfu – is situated 2 cun lateral to the nipple line in the second intercostal space (Figure 2.7). It is known as the master point of the lungs, and as such can be used in the treatment of sports people. Stimulating massage is used during training to tonify the breathing mechanism before a race or any kind of exertion, also afterwards to ease panting, breathlessness or general exhaustion.
    Lu 7 – Lieque – is one of the great points, and is situated 1.5 cun proximal to the transverse wrist crease. As stated before, this point is known as the 'oxygen' point of the lungs and as such is used as a first aid point in revival from exhaustion; it is also useful in asthmatic attacks in the surgery or on the field. It is also a distal point in the treatment of anterior shoulder pain.

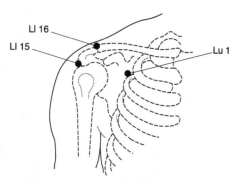

Figure 2.7   Anterior aspect of shoulder showing Lu 1.

The large intestine meridian

LI 1 – Shangyang – is situated medial to the base of the nail on the index finger and is the tsing point of the large intestine meridian. It is used specifically in toothache and pain around the mouth, and is also a revival point in unconsciousness. (Figure 2.6).

LI 4 – Hegu – is situated on the highest point on the mound of the first interosseous muscle with the thumb and forefinger opposed. As stated in the previous section, LI 4 is probably the most commonly used point in acupressure, either in isolation or in tandem with other points. Its very great uses are twofold. It is one of the best 'calming' points and can be used in generalized muscle spasm, tension or anxiety and to calm patients down prior to treatment. It is also used extensively in pain relief to the face, sinuses and anterior aspect of the chest. A truly great point.

LI 11 – Quichi – is located at the lateral edge of the elbow crease when the elbow is flexed. This is used as a local point in the treatment of tennis elbow, also as a general point in calming (sedation) or energizing (stimulation). (Figure 2.6).

LI 15 – Jianyu – is located at the antero-inferior border of the acromio-clavicular joint, inferior to the acromion process when the arm is in adduction. It is a very powerful point and can be used for painful conditions around the neck (anterior and posterior), throat and head, as well as being used as a local point in acromio-clavicular strain and lateral shoulder pain. It is one of the Minor chakra points, is associated with the throat chakra and as such can be used to ease tension and anxiety in the shoulder region and all the way down the arm. (Figure 2.7).

LI 16 – Jugu – is situated in the depression between the acromium and the spine of the scapula. It is again a powerful point, but is not as powerful as LI 15 in that it has more of a defined locally acting role and less of a generally acting one. It is therefore used extensively in the treatment of shoulder, neck and upper limb conditions. (Figure 2.7).

Stomach meridian

St 36 – Sannli – is one of the very great points in acupressure. It is located one finger's breadth lateral to the tibial tubercle and 3 cun below the inferior-lateral aspect of the patella (Figure 2.3). As well as being an excellent local point in knee conditions, it is one of the very great points in energy giving. When given stimulating massage it provides a general energy tonic and can be used in energizing muscles and enhancing performance. It is a very good point for improving muscular tone.

St 38 – Tiaokou – is situated 8 cun below St 35 (Figure 2.3). It is an excellent point for the treatment of shoulder conditions, and is said to be the reflex point of the shoulder. It can be used when there is very acute shoulder pain and it is difficult for the therapist to touch the shoulder. Gentle massage and holding the point can work miracles in releasing lateral shoulder pain, thus allowing movement of the gleno-humeral joint.

The spleen meridian

Sp 4 – Gongsun – is positioned on the medial aspect of the foot in a depression at the anterior and inferior border of the first metatarsal bone. Sp 4 is one of the key points of the eight extraordinary meridians, and has the general use of easing feelings of suffocation and stuffiness. It can also be used as a revival point, and is applied as such in certain martial art procedures. (Figure 2.4).

The heart meridian

Ht 7 – Shenmen – is the only point that is commonly used (Figure 2.5). This is a great point and has been mentioned in the previous section. It is used in cases of anxiety and insomnia.

The small intestine meridian

Si 3 – Houxi – is located at the end of the transverse crease proximal to the fifth metacarpo-phalangeal joint when the hand is clenched. This point is very widely used. It is the key point of the governor meridian (Du mai), and therefore can be considered in most spinal conditions. It has particular uses in the treatment of neck stiffness and low back pain, and is also used as a first aid point in epistaxis (with LI 2). (Figure 2.7).

The bladder meridian

The bladder meridian is perhaps the most used of all the meridians in acupressure. Its significance is that it lies parallel to the spine and also travels down the posterior aspect of the leg. It is therefore used extensively in spinal conditions and sciatica as well as foot problems. The points between Bl 11 and Bl 28 lie along what is called the inner bladder line, situated 1.5 cun lateral to the spinous processes of the dorsal and lumbar spine. These are called associated effect points (Shu), and are used to provide a diagnosis and treatment to the underlying organs. The remaining important points on the bladder meridian are as follows.

Bl 40 – Weizhong – is located in the centre of the popliteal fossa (Figure 2.8). As well as being an excellent point in posterior knee pain, it is used extensively in the treatment of sciatica, low back pain and sacro-iliitis. It is also the knee chakra, and is associated with the elbow chakra (P 3) and also with the base chakra. Using this form of acupressure healing can again be effective in the treatment of low back pain and sciatica.

Bl 57– Chengshan – is located midway between the popliteal crease and the heel (Figure 2.8). It is indicated in the treatment of heel pain, sciatica, and pain in the sole of the foot.

Bl 60 – Kunlun – is located between the posterior border of the external malleolus and the medial aspect of the tendo-achilles at the same level as the tip of the malleolus. It is used extensively in pain relief, especially in the lumbo-sacral area, sciatica and foot. It is, however, one the most used points for relief of pain anywhere. It is said to be the lower limb equivalent of LI 4.

Bl 62 – Shenmai – is located 0.5 cun inferior to the lateral malleolus. It is one of the great points and is very influential in the treatment of pain, especially in the spine and leg.

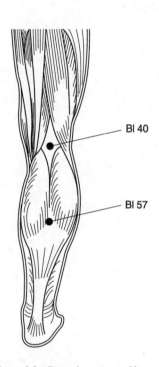

— Bl 40

— Bl 57

Figure 2.8 Posterior aspect of leg showing Bl 40 and Bl 57.

The kidney meridian

Ki 1 – Yongquan – is located in the depression at the junction of the anterior and middle third of the sole in a depression between the second and third metatarso-phalangeal joints (Figure 2.9). This is the only meridian acupressure point on the sole of the foot and it is of vital importance. It is said to be the foot chakra, and hence has much power that can be utilized. It is used in the general balancing of energies (superior and inferior, left and right), in leg length adjustments and in pain relief of the lower spine and leg. It is also used to calm patients if they are in a stressed state, and it is extremely good in anxiety states, especially claustrophobia.

Ki 6 – Zhaohai – is situated 1 cun directly below the tip of the medial malleolus. As stated before, it is one of the great points. Its use in musculo-skeletal conditions is as a distant point in the treatment of adductor/groin strain and in strain of the medial ligament of the knee. Ki 6 is also one the best energy points and is used in meditation and Qi Gong.

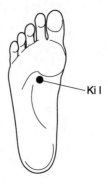

Figure 2.9 Plantar aspect of foot showing Ki 1.

The pericardium meridian

Although there are some powerful points on the pericardium line that can be used in general energy balancing, in particular P 3 (elbow), P 6 (great point – wrist) and P 8 (hand), they are not used as such in musculo-tendinous conditions with the exception of the relief of localized pain.

The three heater meridian

The same is true of the three heater or triple energizer meridian. There are some wonderful points on it that are used in localized conditions and general energy balancing, but none that are specifically used in the treatment of musculo-skeletal conditions.

The gall bladder meridian

As discussed in the first chapter, the gall bladder meridian is part of the Wood element and has a particular affinity for tendons and soft tissue.

GB 20 – Fengchi – is situated between the origins of the sternocleidomastoid and the trapezius muscles. It is an excellent point for the relief of neck tension, cervical pain and torticollis as well as occipital headaches. (See Figure 8.1).

GB 21 – Jianjing – is located midway between the seventh cervical spinous process and the acromium process at the highest point of the shoulder. This is a common trigger point in the treatment of neck tension, muscular spasm and neck pain. Deep pressure to this point helps energize the arm and can be used to heat the arms and hands when they are cold. (See Figure 7.6).

GB 34 – Yanglinguan – is located in the depression anterior and inferior to the head of the fibula. This is possibly the most influential point in tendinous conditions and must be considered in every case of chronic tendinous imbalance. It is also a very good diagnostic point to see if there are any chronic tendon problems – the point will be very tender if there is chronic pain affecting tendons anywhere in the body. (Figure 2.3).

The liver meridian

The liver meridian is the Yin channel of the Wood element, and has a particular affinity for muscle and muscular conditions. It is therefore used extensively in all muscular conditions.

Li 3 – Taichong – is situated 2 cun proximal to the margin of the web between the first and second toes. As previously described, this is a great point, being the source point of the liver. It should be considered in cramp and also in muscular stiffness, wherever in the body it occurs.

Li 8 – Quaquan – is located at the medial end of the transverse crease of the knee joint, in a depression at the anterior border of the semitendinosis and semimembranosis muscles. This point is used extensively in chronic spinal pain and conditions where there is much chronic stiffness. It is also used for cold feet, in combination with St 36. (Figure 2.4).

The governor (Du mai) meridian

As stated in Chapter 1, the governor meridian is used mostly in conjunction with the inner bladder line for treatment to the underlying or associated organs. There are some very important points that can help with treatment of musculo-skeletal and sports injuries.

Gov 2 – Yaoshu – is situated at the junction between the sacrum and the coccyx. This is an extremely important point. It is said to be the posterior aspect of the base (muladhara) chakra, and is significant in *all* spinal conditions. The point is stimulated in chronic conditions and sedated and balanced with other points in acute conditions. This approach will be fully explained elsewhere.

Gov 4 – Mingmen – is located between the spinous processes of L2 and L3. This point has an affinity with kidney energy and the adrenals. It can be used in cases of extreme physical and mental exhaustion or to help an athlete recover from exhaustive exercise. Stimulating massage should be used here. Conversely, when sedated it can be used in calming the system and to prevent the overproduction of cortisol and adrenaline. A very important point!

Gov 11 – Shendao – is located below the spinous process of the fifth dorsal vertebra. This point is directly linked to heart energy and can be used with stimulating massage in fainting and swooning and sudden cerebral anaemia. It raises arterial tension by causing the production of adrenalin. It is one of the master points in certain forms of martial art.

Gov 14 – Daizhui – is situated between the spinous processes of C7 and D1. It is said to be the reunion point for all the Yang meridians, and as such is one of the most influential energy points. It is the posterior aspect of the throat chakra, and has a direct link to the thyroid gland. It can be used with stimulating massage in order to provide instant energy for your athlete or patient.

Gov 18 – Qiangjian – is situated at the junction of the occipital and parietal bones on the mid-line. This point can be massaged to great effect when stamina is needed. It is thought there is a direct link with the hypothalamus. (See Figure 8.2 for all the Governor points mentioned).

The conception (Ren mai) meridian

Con 6 – Qihai – is located 1.5 cun below the umbilicus (Figure 2.10). This is a very important energy point, and relates to the sacral chakra. It is also known as the *hara* point or the Sea of Energy. It is used as a sedative massage in general relaxation and insomnia, also with stimulating massage in order to bring energy to the areas below the point. This can be very useful in most chronic pelvic imbalances and in people who have cold loins and lower limbs. A magic point!

Con 14 – Jujue – is situated 6 cun superior to the umbilicus or just below the xiphoid in people who possess it! (Figure 2.10). This point is said to be directly linked with the solar plexus (coeliac plexus) and as such is a very powerful energy point. It is sedated in agitation and anxiety and stimulated (carefully) to provide energy to the stomach, liver and pancreas. This could be useful with athletes who have a sudden hypoglycaemic experience.

Con 22 – Tiantu – is situated at the centre of the suprasternal fossa 0.5 cun above the sternal notch (Figure 2.10). This point is said directly to influence the thyroid gland and is the anterior point that represents the throat chakra. It is therefore a very important energy point and can be used in patients who are depleted of energy and stamina and who are prone to overweight and osteoarthritic changes.

Non-meridian (extra) points

Extra 1 – Yintang – is situated between the medial end of the two eyebrows. This point is said to be the anterior aspect of the ajna (brow) chakra and as such is a very important point. It is said to have an influence directly on the pituitary gland and is one of our very best points in sedation to relax the person. Never stimulate this point!!

There is a special point between C3 and C4. There is not an official name for this point, but the author has used it for several years to good effect in the treatment of both rheumatoid and osteoarthritis. This point is generally stimulated as it is used more often than not in chronic osteoarthritic conditions.

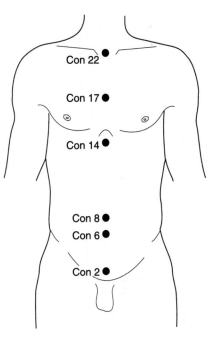

Figure 2.10 Anterior chest and abdomen showing Con 6, Con 14 and Con 22.

3
Zones, reflexes and chakras

Zones

Although the use and practice with energy zones has lasted as long as acupressure and has its roots firmly entrenched in traditional Oriental medicine, the modern practice of 'zone therapy' began with an American ENT specialist, Dr William Fitzgerald. Dr Fitzgerald noticed that his patients varied in the amount of pain that they suffered post-operatively. He discovered that patients who had performed their own kind of acupressure or 'painful point therapy' faired better than those patients who were ignorant of such procedures. He researched this at length and discovered that the human body can be divided into ten equal sections (five on each side of the body) along its vertical plane from head to feet. These sections are not just on the skin, but appeared to affect the underlying organs as well. An American masseuse, Eunice Ingham, was interested in Dr Fitzgerald's work, and she concentrated her efforts in mapping out both vertical and horizontal zones on the feet as opposed to using body points. She invented what is a major philosophy of reflexology, namely foot zonal therapy.

In the beginning zone therapy concentrated on the joints, mainly of the hands and feet, with the use of heavy pressure lasting up to a few minutes in duration. It has since evolved to become the most used form of reflex therapy in the Western world.

Zone therapy is a system of healing that connects the different body sections using invisible dividing lines. The division of ten vertical zones is due to the number of fingers and toes. As shown in Figure 3.1, the thumb and the great toe together with the medial fifth of the body are in the most medial zone, whereas the little toe and little finger together with the most lateral part of the body are in the lateral zone. The other three zones are placed equally between these two. Each section includes the inside of the body from front to back; therefore the reflex points on the different zones are found in the front as well as on the back. Eunice Ingham maintained that a tension in any section affects the section along the full body length – like a blocked stream, it causes a state of surplus

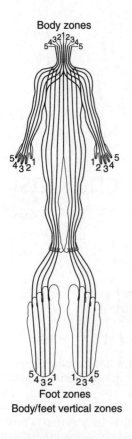

Body zones

Foot zones
Body/feet vertical zones

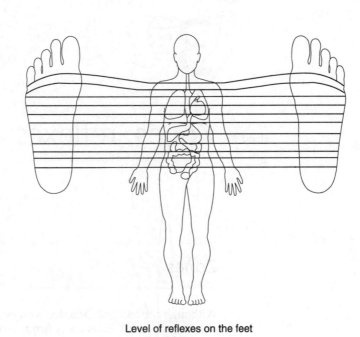

Level of reflexes on the feet

Figure 3.1 Level of reflexes on the feet.

before the blockage and a shortage immediately behind it. In a similar way, the body will be affected by a blockage in any part; it will cause a problem in front of and behind the blockage, and also affects the section as a whole. Areas of great sensitivity, callousity and tension in the reflexes on the feet (or body) indicate a problematic section of the body and its location. This principle can be used when placing direct pressure on any point within the section – it will affect the whole zone.

In addition to the vertical division, zone therapy uses horizontal divisions (as shown in Figure 3.1). This is a very useful way of dividing the body up into treatable sections on the feet.

Yet another system within the discipline known as zone therapy is known as 'parallel zones'. In simple terms, if it is impossible to treat a part of the body locally, due to an open wound or some other contraindicating disease factor, its parallel area can be treated. The main connections are that the hand is parallel to the foot, the knee is parallel to the elbow, the shoulder is parallel to the hip and the pelvis is parallel to the neck (Figures 3.2 and 3.3). This can be broken down further; the thumb is parallel (and is therefore reflected) to the great toe, the little finger is parallel to the little toe, the top of the neck is parallel with the base of the spine, and so on. There are profound implications in this type of acupressure philosophy for the way musculo-skeletal conditions can be treated. Please remember, at this very early stage of the book, that each and every part of the body – be it joint, muscle or tendon – has one or more reflected areas (reflexes) that can be used to treat the injured part. Furthermore, whenever there is an injured part of the

Figure 3.2   Parallel zones: hand with foot; elbow with knee.

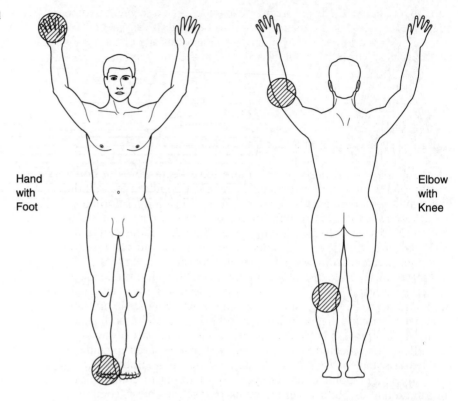

Hand
with
Foot

Elbow
with
Knee

Figure 3.3   Parallel zones: shoulder with hip; neck with pelvis.

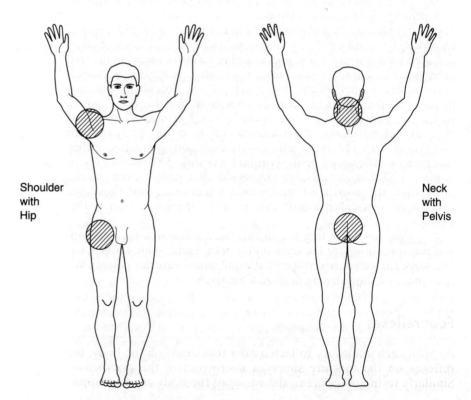

Shoulder
with
Hip

Neck
with
Pelvis

body to be treated, there will *always* be a tender area elsewhere both to guide the therapist in the diagnosis and to be used in treatment. This type of zone therapy is very similar to the associations of the minor chakra points, which will be discussed later in the chapter.

Reflexes

As the reader is obviously aware, there have been scores of books written on the subject of reflexology. The most popular type and the one that is most practised is, of course, foot reflexology. Information about foot reflexology is available in many notable tomes, so it is prudent in this book just to mention the reflexes on the foot as part of the whole picture of reflexes that appear on the body and can be used especially when treating musculo-skeletal conditions. There are several different separate disciplines and philosophies within reflexology (a better 'holistic' word is reflextherapy) that will be mentioned. Some are obviously more important than others, and some are only used in analysis and diagnosis whereas others are used for both analysis and treatment. As has been stated before, every part of the body has reflexes or reflected points or areas that can be used to guide us in diagnosis and for treatment of the dis-eased part. Each reflected area and tender point is the body's way of trying to communicate information to us. Reflexes are to be used as subtle energy communicators, and should be treated as such. They should never be massaged or touched in a harsh or violent way!!!

It is considered that there are as many as 14 reflected areas in the body that can be used for diagnosis and ten reflected areas that are used for treatment. The areas of diagnosis are found in the iris, face, tongue, teeth, temple, pulse, hand, skull, ear, foot, abdomen (two different ones), spine (several) and the so called 'listening posts'. The areas that are used in treatment are the skull, hands, feet, face, abdomen, ears and spine, as well as major and minor chakras and meridians. There are also points on the body that are associated with the lymphatic circulation and are called either Chapman's reflexes or neuro-lymphatic points. The philosophy of applied kinesiology has also suggested that points exist on the body that are associated with blood circulation, and these are called neuro-vascular points. These will be discussed later in this chapter.

The reflected areas that are mainly used when treating musculo-skeletal conditions are the ones on the foot, hand, skull, temple, ear and spine (as well as neuro-lymphatic and neuro-vascular points). We shall mention the listening posts in Chapter 6.

Foot reflexes

As with each and every reflected area that exists on the body, the reflexes on the foot are simply a microcosm of the macrocosm. Similarly to the other areas, the whole of the body can be mapped out on the feet. Foot reflextherapy has its roots in traditional Oriental medicine, and its use as a treatment modality has stood the test of time over thousands of years. There have been many types of foot reflexology devised and practised, including zone therapy in isolation, a mixture of zone therapy and organic placement massage, symptomatic reflexology (where just the symptoms are treated), holistic reflexology (where the organs of excretion are treated firstly followed by areas that would create a balance of the whole), light touch reflexology, treating the reflected chakra points, metamorphic technique.....the list goes on. There are also several schools of thought regarding the amount of pressure that the practitioner uses in treatment, ranging from hardly touching the point or area to virtually boring a hole into the flesh. It all depends on the practitioner's philosophy! It is very important to have an open mind on the issue and not to denigrate another approach simply because it is not the way that you do it! There is a parallel here in the different types and techniques of acupuncture. There is a place for all of them (yes – symptomatic pin pricking sometimes works!!). The author has known of wonderful cures using the harshest of approaches, where the therapist spent minutes in attempting to break down the 'crystals', having the patient hovering halfway between the couch and the ceiling; and also of the opposite, where the therapist used the very gentle approach or did not touch the skin at all. The author's personal preference is widely known by his students and patients alike – a reflex point is to be respected!!! It should not be treated harshly, but rather be used as a signal as to the cause of the imbalance. Having used most methods of reflexology over nearly 30 years in practice, there is no doubt that, personally, the author believes the gentle approach is the most useful and effective. It also creates far less post-treatment trauma and aggravation.

The areas on the feet that are useful in the treatment of musculo-skeletal conditions are as follows.

The spine is reflected along the antero-medial aspect of the feet. Please note that the prominence of the cervico-dorsal junction is reflected at the distal end of the first metatarsal (see Figures 3.4, 3.5 and 3.6).

The peripheral joints are reflected along the lateral aspects of the feet (see Figure 3.7), with an additional area for the hip joint reflected underneath the medial malleolus.

The main muscles of the body are reflected as shown in Figures 3.8, 3.9, 3.10 and 3.11. These areas can be very helpful to ease acute muscular soreness and also as an aid in helping with the pain of chronic muscle imbalance. As has been mentioned before, when there is an injured part of the body, the associated reflex will become tender. The more chronic the problem and the more in need of treatment the part is, the more tender will be its reflex. Therefore, when diagnosing musculo-skeletal imbalance via the feet or any of the other reflected areas, the priority of treatment lies with the most tender point, regardless of what the patient may be complaining of symptomatically!! If this rule is obeyed, some surprising results will ensue!

When it comes to treatment via the foot reflexes, it all depends what type of musculo-skeletal condition is being treated and whether

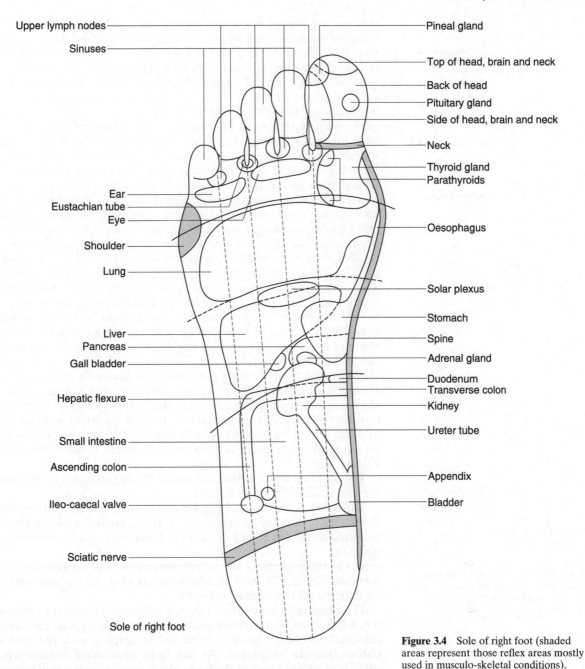

Upper lymph nodes
Sinuses
Ear
Eustachian tube
Eye
Shoulder
Lung
Liver
Pancreas
Gall bladder
Hepatic flexure
Small intestine
Ascending colon
Ileo-caecal valve
Sciatic nerve

Pineal gland
Top of head, brain and neck
Back of head
Pituitary gland
Side of head, brain and neck
Neck
Thyroid gland
Parathyroids
Oesophagus
Solar plexus
Stomach
Spine
Adrenal gland
Duodenum
Transverse colon
Kidney
Ureter tube
Appendix
Bladder

Sole of right foot

Figure 3.4 Sole of right foot (shaded areas represent those reflex areas mostly used in musculo-skeletal conditions).

or not it is acute or chronic. In acute conditions, it is often just enough to place the finger on the associated reflex point and hold it until the pain eases. It also helps if a finger of one hand can be placed on the acutely painful area of the body and the same finger of the other hand on the associated reflex – this seems to augment the treatment and is a much more satisfactory way of relieving pain and easing localized muscular spasm to the area. In cases of muscular and joint stiffness, and in any situation where there is a long-standing injury, the reflected area(s) on the feet should be *gently* massaged until the patient

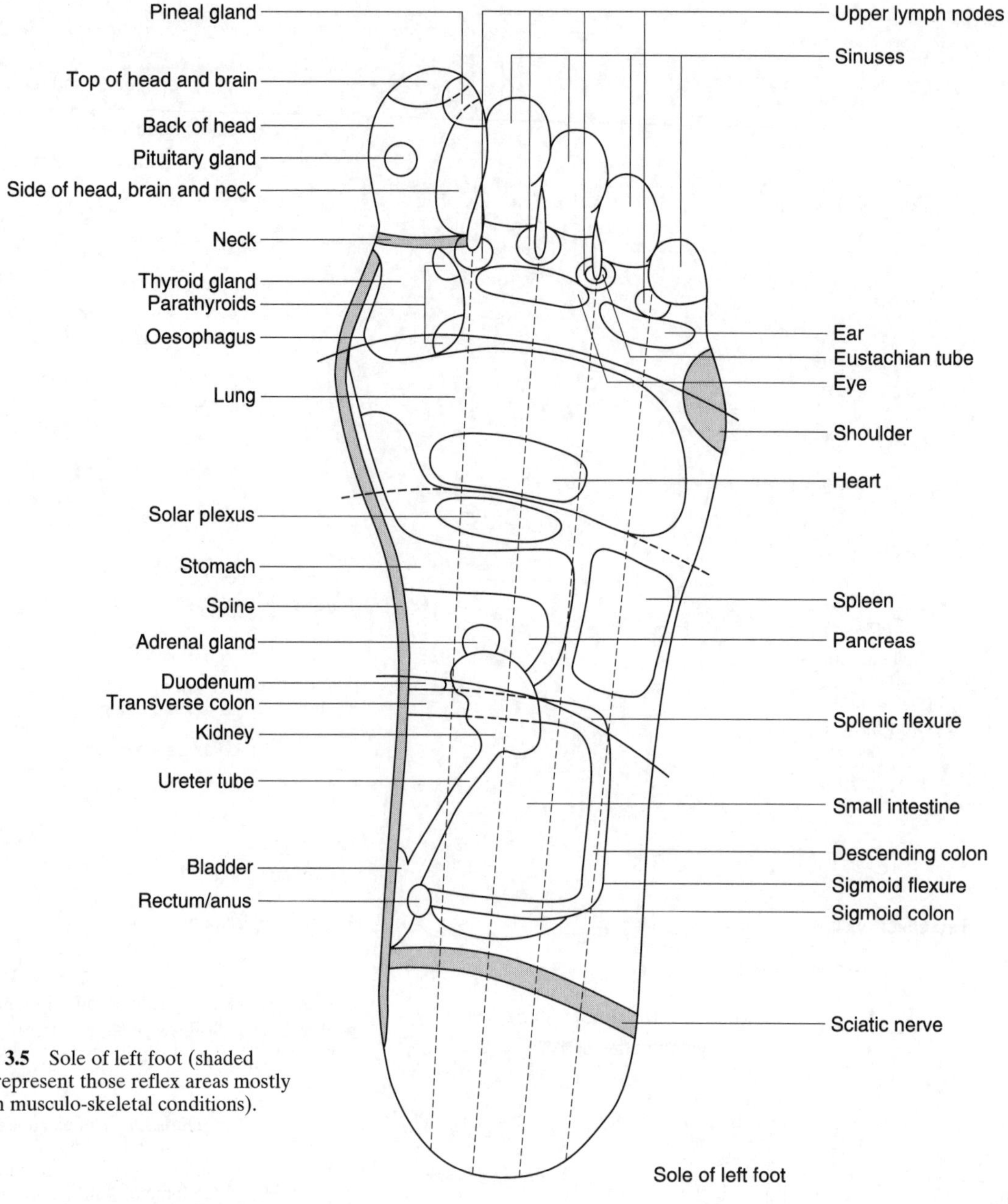

Pineal gland
Top of head and brain
Back of head
Pituitary gland
Side of head, brain and neck
Neck
Thyroid gland
Parathyroids
Oesophagus
Lung
Solar plexus
Stomach
Spine
Adrenal gland
Duodenum
Transverse colon
Kidney
Ureter tube
Bladder
Rectum/anus

Upper lymph nodes
Sinuses
Ear
Eustachian tube
Eye
Shoulder
Heart
Spleen
Pancreas
Splenic flexure
Small intestine
Descending colon
Sigmoid flexure
Sigmoid colon
Sciatic nerve

Sole of left foot

Figure 3.5 Sole of left foot (shaded areas represent those reflex areas mostly used in musculo-skeletal conditions).

informs the practitioner that the area feels more relaxed. This could be performed as long as 10 minutes prior to the main treatment, and is a good way of commencing the treatment. It would be helpful, though, if the reader is not familiar with the practice of foot reflexology, to try and learn this noble art in more detail. It is not sufficient simply to ease discomfort in the associated areas of the body. A more holistic attitude is always necessary – for example, massage of the large intestine reflex in all cases of chronic low back pain in an attempt to ease the sluggishness of the bowel and hence the lower

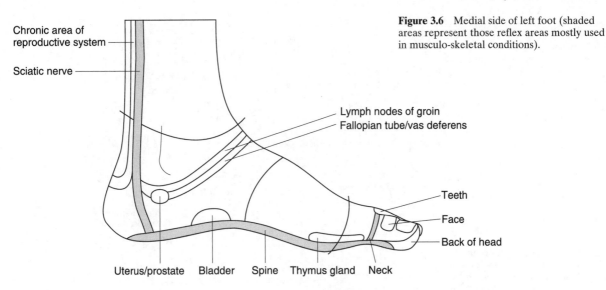

Figure 3.6 Medial side of left foot (shaded areas represent those reflex areas mostly used in musculo-skeletal conditions).

Chronic area of reproductive system

Sciatic nerve

Lymph nodes of groin
Fallopian tube/vas deferens

Teeth
Face
Back of head

Uterus/prostate   Bladder   Spine   Thymus gland   Neck

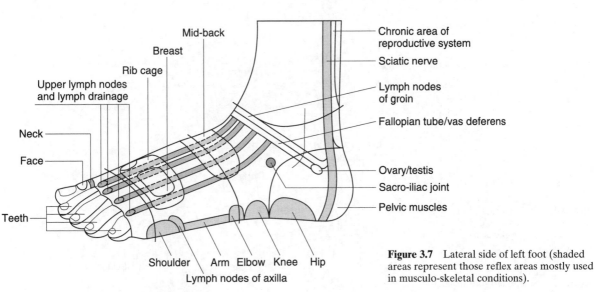

Mid-back
Breast
Rib cage
Upper lymph nodes and lymph drainage
Neck
Face
Teeth

Chronic area of reproductive system
Sciatic nerve
Lymph nodes of groin
Fallopian tube/vas deferens
Ovary/testis
Sacro-iliac joint
Pelvic muscles

Shoulder   Arm   Elbow   Knee   Hip
Lymph nodes of axilla

Figure 3.7 Lateral side of left foot (shaded areas represent those reflex areas mostly used in musculo-skeletal conditions).

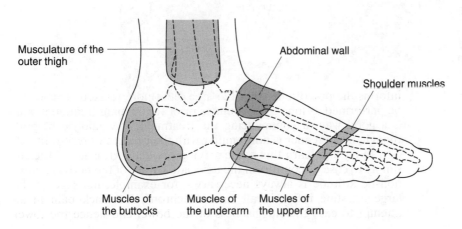

Figure 3.8 Reflex zones of the musculature of the body: shoulder, upper arm, underarm, abdominal wall, buttocks, outer thigh.

Musculature of the outer thigh

Abdominal wall

Shoulder muscles

Muscles of the buttocks   Muscles of the underarm   Muscles of the upper arm

Figure 3.9   Reflex zones of the musculature of the body, inner foot: ribs, pelvis, inner thigh.

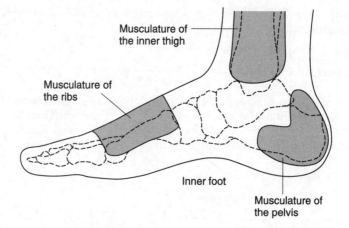

Musculature of the inner thigh

Musculature of the ribs

Inner foot

Musculature of the pelvis

Figure 3.10   Reflex zones of the musculature of the body, outer foot: ribs, musculature between ribs and hips.

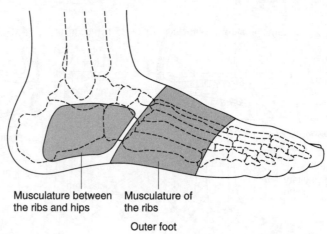

Musculature between the ribs and hips   Musculature of the ribs

Outer foot

Figure 3.11   Reflex zones of the musculature of the body, dorsal view of feet: shoulder, upper arm, underarm, ribs.

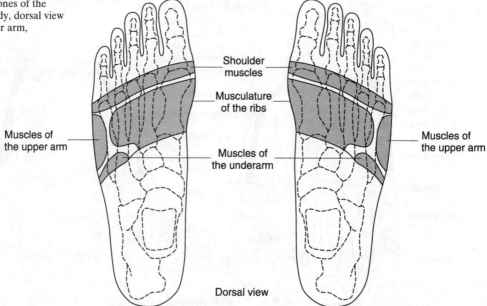

Shoulder muscles

Musculature of the ribs

Muscles of the upper arm

Muscles of the underarm

Muscles of the upper arm

Dorsal view

lumbar spine. Care must also be taken in massaging the reflexes of the lymphatics, especially in chronic conditions.

Hand reflexes

Hand reflexology is not as popular as its foot counterpart, and some would say that it is not as powerful or as effective. As shown in Figure 3.12, the whole of the body can be mapped out on the hands. Generally speaking, the organs and everything on the anterior aspect

Figure 3.12 Hand reflexes (shaded areas represent those reflex areas mostly used in musculo-skeletal conditions).

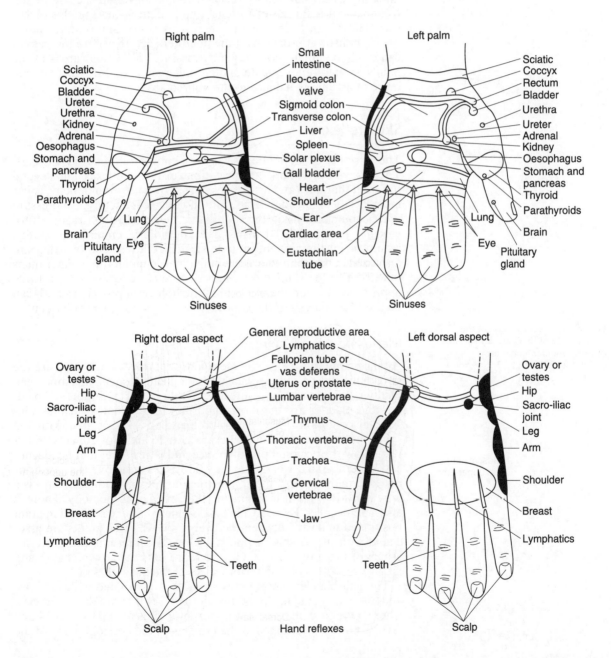

Hand reflexes

of the body lie on the palmar aspect of the hands, whereas the joints and bones lie on the dorsal aspect. The spine is located along the lateral aspect of the thumb, and the peripheral joints of the hip, elbow and shoulder lie on the medial aspect of the little finger, in exactly the same positions as they would be expected to be found on the feet.

As with the feet, the reflexes on the hand will be tender if the associated part of the body is in a state of imbalance and needs treatment. The reflexes on the hand, though, will not exhibit the same degree of acute tenderness as the ones on the feet, because the hands are in everyday use much more than the feet and therefore reflexes become 'hidden'. The great beauty of hand reflexology is in the use of self treatment. It is far easier to teach the patient to massage his or her own hands than to massage the feet. It is not so important to introduce a holistic approach with the hand reflexes; therefore the patient can easily be taught how to gently massage the various areas of the hands, how to relieve acute and chronic pain and also how to create more of an energy balance to the injured area.

Skull reflexes

The existence of skull reflexes has been known for thousands of years. There have been many interpretations of these reflexes, and several different therapies and disciplines have grown up around them. These include Tibetan head massage, phrenology acupuncture, acupressure and acupuncture using the meridians, Indian head massage, neuro-vascular points as used in applied kinesiology, cranial osteopathy, cranio-sacral therapy and muscle stretch reflexes. The two that are discussed in this chapter are the individual acupoints on the meridians that traverse the skull and the muscle stretch reflexes. Both of these approaches are very helpful within the holistic approach, as both can be used for analysis of the condition and for subsequent treatment.

Meridians and acupoints

As shown in Figure 3.13, the meridians that traverse the skull are the governor, conception, stomach, triple heater, small intestine, gall bladder, bladder and large intestine. Of these, the governor, gall bladder and bladder are the most important in the context of musculo-skeletal conditions. The governor meridian is associated with the spine, and the most useful points are Gov 16 and Gov 20. Gov 16 lies just below the occipital protuberance and is very useful in headaches and general spinal weakness. Gov 20 lies 7 cun above the posterior hairline, midway on a line connecting the apex of both ears. This is a very important point in balancing the energies of the body. There is also a point called Extra 1 (Yin tang), which is an extra meridian point positioned midway between the eyebrows. All three points are associated with major chakra points – Gov 16 represents the posterior aspect of the brow chakra, Gov 20 represents the crown chakra and Extra 1 represents the anterior aspect of the brow chakra.

The gall bladder meridian as a whole is associated with tendons, and there are some useful points on the body that are discussed elsewhere. On the skull, the most important points are GB 7, GB 14 and GB 20. GB 7 is positioned at the crossing of the horizontal line of the

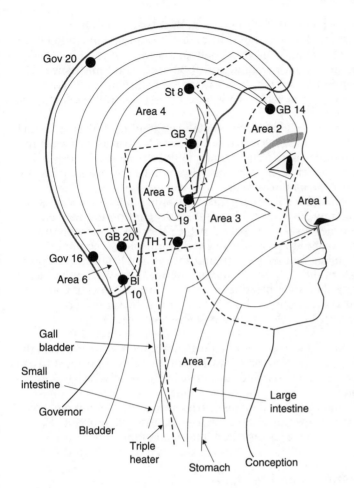

Figure 3.13 Reflex areas of the head.

Area 1. Nose diseases
Area 2. Eye diseases
Area 3. Cheek, tooth,
lip diseases
Area 4. Head, face,
eye, nose,
temporal region,
occipital region diseases
Area 5. Ear diseases
Area 6. Eye, nose, head,
neck, tongue, ear diseases
Area 7. Neck, throat,
tongue diseases

auricle and the line that projects from the anterior auricle, on the temple. This point is widely used in cranio-sacral therapy as a listening post point, and as such can be used within the philosophy of acupressure for a similar purpose. This will be explained in Chapter 6. GB 14 is positioned 1 cun above the midpoint of the eyebrow and, as well as being useful in frontal headaches, it is a very useful point for general relaxation prior to the main treatment. GB 20 is positioned in a depression between the sternocleidomastoid muscle and the upper portion of the trapezius muscle, directly inferior to the occipital protuberance. It is useful as a local point, gently pressed or massaged, in the treatment of occipital headaches. It is also of vital significance in atlas bone imbalance, which will be dealt with in Chapter 8.

The stomach meridian commences in two points on the face. These two points have changed their number over the past few years; St 1 was where St 8 is now, and it is this point that is the most significant. It is situated 0.5 cun within the anterior hairline at the corner of the forehead. As well as being a most useful local point for frontal headaches, especially when caused by toxic or cold food hitting the stomach, it is also another one of our listening post points. It governs the general condition of soft tissue (explained later).

There is just one significant point on the bladder meridian, at Bl 10. This is situated 1.5 cun lateral to Gov 15 on the lateral side of the trapezius. This point is used in conjunction with GB 20 for occipital headache, and also for treatment of occipito-atlanto imbalance. The bladder meridian as a whole is associated with bone and the spine, and Bl 10 can also be used as a listening post point (although not the best one) for this.

On the triple heater meridian, the most influential acupressure point is TH 17, which is located posterior to the ear-lobe in a depression between the angle of the mandible and the mastoid process. It is used as a minor chakra point and also as a listening post point for imbalance of the hypothalamus.

On the small intestine meridian there is just one point that is significant; namely Si 19 which, being the last point on this meridian, is situated in the depression between the tragus and the mandibular joint when the mouth is slightly opened. Locally it can be used for tinnitus and otalgia, but its great significance is as a listening post point for the state of the tempero-mandibular joint. There are no significant points along the large intestine and the conception vessels found on the skull that are useful in the treatment of physical injuries.

To summarize the uses of meridian points on the skull:

1. They can be used as listening post points in order to ascertain the energic quality of areas of systems of the body. This most useful adjunct to analysis and diagnosis will be discussed fully in Chapter 5.
2. They can be used as diagnostic trigger points for either local pain or imbalance within the meridian or its associated organ.
3. They can be used as localized treatment points.

Stretch reflexes on the skull

This particular approach forms part of the applied kinesiology philosophy, which was devised by American chiropractors in the early 1960s. It is an extremely useful tool, and should be taught and used more than it is at present. As with all reflected areas, the whole of the body can be mapped out on the skull. However, as opposed to other reflected areas, this discipline deals entirely with the muscular structure of the body; hence its great value in the treatment of musculo-skeletal conditions. Chapter 5 deals with the applied kinesiological paradigm of being able to strengthen weak muscles, but by using stretch reflexes, tension, pain and stiffness can be eased both in acutely sore muscles and in chronically affected ones. The great strength of the stretch reflexes is in the treatment of chronic muscular imbalance; for example, easing the tension in the erector spinae muscle in chronic spinal complaints. It should always be used at the beginning of the treatment. Unlike the other reflected areas, there is not much localized tenderness with the reflex, and the practitioner has to know where the reflex is. The ones that are used in everyday practice just have to be learnt!! These include the erector spinae, quadriceps, hamstrings, abdominals, biceps, deltoids and gastrocnemius. The practice is relatively easy. When there is a muscular imbalance – for example, a weak quadriceps following a meniscectomy operation – the pads of

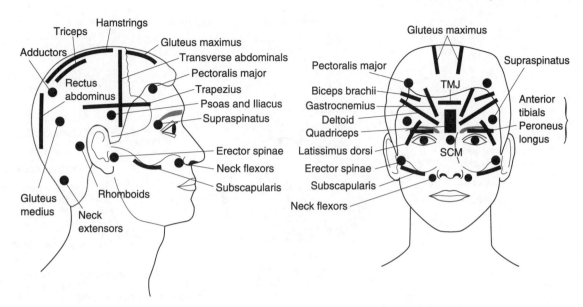

Figure 3.14   Stretch reflexes on the scalp with muscle association.

the opposing fingers are placed *gently* on the reflex and simply held there for about half a minute until a warmth is felt. A slight stretching movement is then given, very subtly, attempting to part the fingers of each hand from each other but not actually moving the fingers on the patient's skin. After about another minute extreme warmth comes to the area, with a feeling of relaxation in the tissues. When this has happened, the treatment is completed and the practitioner can proceed to another type of acupressure, possibly balancing the quadriceps via the acupressure holding points. Alternatively, the hold can be kept on for much longer – the more chronic the condition, the more of a hold is needed for the best results.

Note that there is a non-muscular reflex – the temporo-mandibular joint. This point is of extreme value in the relaxation of the joint prior to its manipulation. As with all forms of acupressure, this is a skill that has to be repeated over and over again until the correct subtlety of approach is achieved. Do not be disappointed if absolutely nothing happens after the first venture into this approach; practice makes perfect!!!

Temporo-sphenoidal line

This is another 'invention' of the American chiropractors who have perfected the applications of applied kinesiology so successfully. In their texts on the subject it is stated that this line (the TS line) is used for analysis and diagnosis only, but there can also be a treatment benefit. The TS line is the suture line that delineates the temporal bone, and it can be easily palpated. Along this line there exist several points that can exhibit tenderness. Applied kinesiology states that each of the tender points along this line is associated with a muscle; this may be so, but in practice it is found that the stretch reflexes previously described have much more of an influence than the TS line on the muscles. The author has given each of the tender points an association

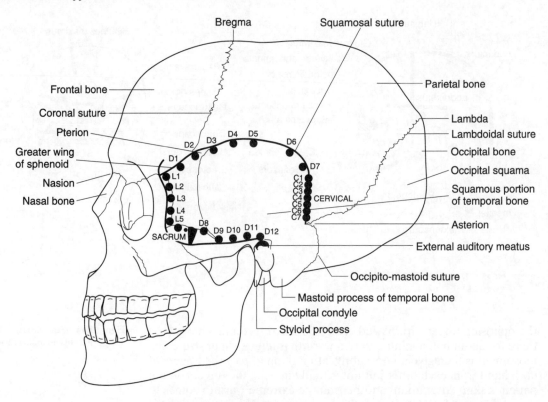

Figure 3.15   Skull – lateral view showing temporo-sphenoidal line.

with the vertebral levels in order that they may be used for both diagnostic and treatment purposes.

Figure 3.15 shows the various vertebral levels reflected upon the TS line in a fairly logical order; the cervicals lumped together at the posterior end of the line, the lumbar spine at the anterior end and the dorsal spine spanning the superior and inferior borders. With the patient lying supine and the practitioner seated behind, the middle fingers of both hands are placed gently along the TS line, commencing and finishing where the practitioner wishes. Exquisite discomfort upon gentle palpation shows there is discomfort and imbalance on the particular vertebra, whereas discomfort on deeper palpation shows that there is a chronic imbalance in the associated vertebral level. Furthermore, if the right-hand side is tender and the left-hand side is not, this shows that the lesion is on the right-hand side of the vertebrae. This could, of course, mean anything, but at least it gives the practitioner an opening gambit towards analysis of the spinal condition. This can be supplemented by all the other reflected pathways, along with orthodox diagnostic methods. When the patient has confirmed all the tender spots, these can either be written down to add to all the other data or they can be used for treatment purposes. In acute lesions of the spine (muscular, ligamentous, disc lesions, subluxation etc.) it is merely sufficient to hold these points with the pads of the middle fingers or any of the other fingers with which you feel comfortable (not the thumbs) until there is a warmth felt under the fingers. The patient will comment that there is a pleasant sensation both in the head and in the part of the spine that is being affected. The hold can be for up to 5 minutes, or for as long as the patient and practitioner are comfortable and the sensation appears to be harmonious. (Sensations will be discussed in Chapter 4.)

In the treatment of chronic lesions of the spine, it is necessary to instigate some gentle massage on the point(s) before the fingers are kept still as above. The point needs to be massaged or stimulated quite a number of times according to the chronicity of the lesion. With very chronic lesions – i.e. over 10 years duration – the points may be alternatively stimulated and held for anything up to 10 minutes before the vertebral level is affected. With the knowledge of the various meridian skull points, stretch reflexes and the TS line, it is obviously apparent to the reader how powerful the skull can be as a tool in the treatment of musculo-skeletal conditions. Indeed, the practitioner may decide to specialize in this approach alone and could spend the majority of a treatment session on treating the spine or peripheral condition just by working on the skull.

Again it is emphasized that practice makes perfect, and it may take several sessions with the use of many 'guinea pig' patients before skills are honed to the level of expertise that is required to give an effective and comfortable treatment.

Ear reflexes

The art of using the ear for treatment, either with needles (auriculotherapy) or with touch, is part of traditional Chinese medicine, and as such has a history as long as traditional Chinese acupuncture. The ear can be used as a reflected area for both diagnosis and treatment. As with all the reflected areas and pathways on the body, the whole of the body can be mapped within the ear. Although the art of auriculotherapy dates back centuries, it was first recognized as a reflex system by Paul Nogier in the 1950s.

As with the other reflected areas in the body, the ear can be used as a signal that there is imbalance elsewhere. The reflected point in the ear can be inflamed, raised, swollen or pitted, depending upon the condition. In general terms, the more chronic the condition, the more microtrophic changes appear in the ear; the more acute the condition, the more red and sensitive the reflex is. Care has to be taken that the reflex is palpated gently and not 'poked about' too much. With experience, the author has found that ear acupressure tends to be most effective when treating acute conditions rather than chronic ones.

Anatomy of the ear

The ear reflexes are said to represent an inverted foetus, with the head being in the lobe, the internal organs being 'protected' within the concha and the limbs and spine being around the scaphoid fossa. For the purposes of using the ear reflexes in treating the musculo-skeletal system, at the very top of the scaphoid fossa is the foot and ankle, fingers and wrist, with the knee and elbow being slightly inferior (Figure 3.16). Although there are some excellent auricular charts for sale, it is impossible for the therapist to find points with any accuracy merely by using a chart. It is important that the therapist looks at the ear before tentatively feeling the general area where an acutely tender area may be felt.

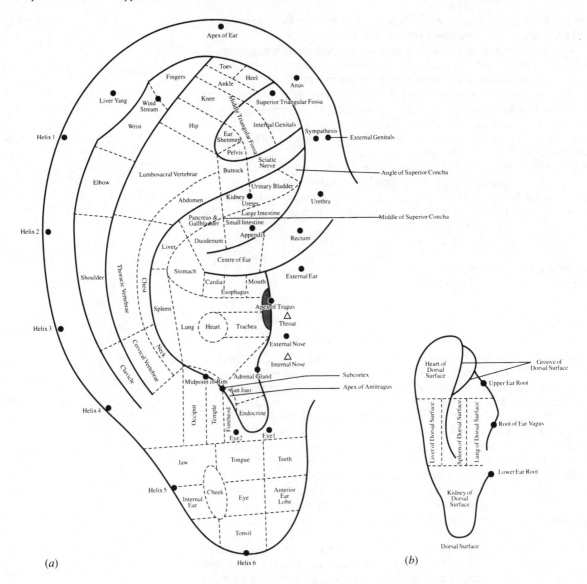

Figure 3.16   Ear reflexes.

Treatment

Once the reflected tender point is found, the therapist may use either the pad of the little finger or a cotton bud to exert a little pressure on the point in order to effect pain relief in the affected part. This technique may last a few minutes. It may be wise to introduce some gentle movement to initiate the healing response, but once the patient's discomfort starts to ease, the finger or cotton bud should be kept perfectly still.

The author's introduction to ear acupressure was at an athletics meeting at Crystal Palace some 25 years ago, in a match between Britain and the Soviet Union. Being confronted by a Soviet athlete with acute pain in the right knee and due on the track for the 400-m hurdles in 10 minutes, speed was of the essence. Very sparse knowledge of ear acupressure came in handy and, having pressed the 'knee' point in the athlete's right ear for 5 minutes combined with 'local' points around the knee, she reported that all the pain had disappeared and it seemed to be an instant success. The athlete competed and won the race. There had been no dialogue, as neither spoke the other's language. In hindsight, it must have been very strange for her to have a foreigner stick a finger in her ear after she complained of knee pain! The story made the popular press, and there seemed to be a great deal of interest at the time.

Reflexes of the spine

Assessment, analysis and treatment of spinal conditions are probably the most common things that physical therapists do. The orthodox therapist is used to dealing with referred pain, parasthesia, dermatomes, sclerotomes and myotomes, but there are several 'energy'-based considerations to take into account. Without a doubt the spinal reflexes are the most useful, but they are regrettably the most complicated to learn and understand. The problem is that there are so many different types of reflexes, based upon many philosophies. The ones that are the most useful in the treatment of musculo-skeletal conditions are as follows:

1. Back transporting points
2. Lovett Brother
3. Muscular associations
4. Occipito-sacral associations
5. Major spinal chakras
6. Organic associations.

There is a whole section dedicated to the many 'relationships' of the spine in Chapter 5, so just one aspect under the umbrella of 'reflexes', namely the back transporting points, is discussed here.

The back transporting points or associated effect points

These points have their derivation in traditional Chinese medicine, and are usually used with acupuncture. They can, however, prove a valuable asset when used with acupressure. They lie on the inner bladder line, which is situated 1.5 cun lateral to the spinous processes (Figure 3.17), and become tender when the associated organ is in a state of stress. The more acutely sick the organ, the more tender the point. They can be of use in two different ways:

1. As reflex points (diagnostic or treatment) to help support the energic quality and quantity of the underlying and associated internal organ. For example, Bl 23 (which is situated 1.5 cun lateral to the space between the spinous processes of L2–3) is associated with the kidneys. This points will be tender if there is any acute kidney imbalance, or if there is any imbalance with the adrenal glands. It will also be tender to a deeper palpation with any chronic kidney imbalance. The usual rules of acupressure apply in treatment; that is, sedation for acute conditions and stimulation for chronic conditions.

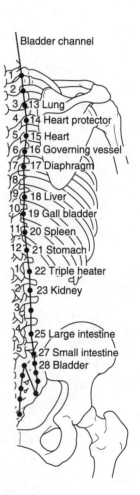

Figure 3.17 The back transporting points.

2. As local points for spinal conditions. For example, Bl 25 (situated between L4–5) might be treated in conditions of these vertebrae, either acute or chronic.

Chakras

It is said that the human frame consists of an interpenetrating series of body forms of different vibrational frequencies, ranging from the physical to the spiritual, with the higher spiritual and mental frequency forms determining the state of the physical body. The appreciation of the existence of our subtle bodies is the bedrock of understanding subtle body healing. The subtle bodies in ascending order out from the physical body are etheric, emotional, mental, intuitional, monadic and divine. The chakras are considered to be force centres or whorls of energy situated at a particular point on the physical body and permeating through the layers of the etheric, emotional and so on in an ever-increasing fan-shaped formation. They are rotating vortices of subtle matter, and are considered to be the focal points for the transmission and reception of energies. The word *chakra* means 'wheel'. A clairvoyant can easily see these energy centres. Each is different in form, colour and energy vibration. There are said to be seven major chakras and 21 minor chakras. The minor chakras are said to be reflected points of the majors, and do not extend any further than the etheric body outwards.

Figure 3.18   Major and minor chakra energy centres.

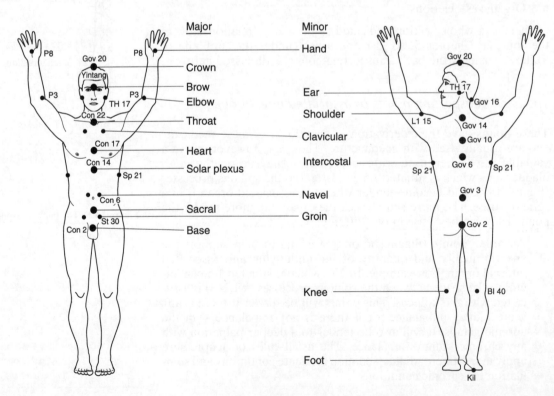

Table 3.1 The major chakras and their levels

Chakra	Spinal level	Ventral level
1. Crown	–	Top of head at point Gov 20
2. Brow	Occipito-atlas junction (Gov 16)	Between the eyes (Extra point 1 – Yintang)
3. Throat	C7–T1 junction (Gov 14)	The sternal notch (Con 22)
4. Heart	T6–T7 junction (Gov 10)	Mid-sternum (Con 17)
5. Solar plexus	T12–L1 junction (Gov 6)	Below xiphoid process (Con 14)
6. Sacral	L4–L5 junction (Gov 3)	Three fingers' width below umbilicus (Con 6)
7. Base	Sacro-coccyx junction (Gov 2)	Symphysis pubis (Con 2)

What the author has attempted to do in teaching this esoteric philosophy to others is to make it 'therapist friendly' and try and take the mystique out of it. These force centres have hitherto been used extensively in yoga, meditation and some of the martial arts, but they can also be used with great effectiveness in hands-on therapy (Figure 3.18).

Table 3.2 The chakras and their associations

Chakra	Coupled minor chakra(s)	Endocrine gland	Organs	Meridian(s)	Spinal level covered	Muscles
1. Crown	Hand and foot	Pineal	Upper brain, right eye	Three heater	Cranium	Trapezius, supraspinatus, facial muscles
2. Brow	Clavicular and groin	Pituitary	Nervous system, ears, nose, left eye	Gall bladder	Cranial base to C4	Anterior and posterior neck muscles
3. Throat	Shoulder and navel	Thyroid	Bronchial organs, lungs, large bowel	Large intestine and lung	C5–T3	Latissimus dorsi, pectorals, triceps
4. Heart	Ear and intercostal	Thymus	Heart, circulation, vagus nerve	Heart and small intestine	T4–T8	Erector spinae
5. Solar plexus	Spleen	Pancreas	Stomach, liver, spleen	Liver and stomach	T9–L2	Abdominals, quadriceps
6. Sacral	Spleen	Gonads	Reproductive system, fluid balance	Spleen and pericardium	L3–S2	Hamstrings, anterior tibials
7. Base	Elbow and knee	Adrenals	Spinal column, kidney	Bladder and kidney	S3 to coccyx	Psoas, soleus, gastrocnemius and foot muscles

Table 3.3   Associations of the minor chakras

Minor chakra	Coupled minor	Coupled major	Anatomical position	Acupuncture point
Foot	Hand	Crown	Sole of foot	Ki 1
Hand	Foot	Crown	Palm of hand	P 8
Knee	Elbow	Base	Popliteal fossa	Bl 40
Elbow	Knee	Base	Cubital fossa	P 3
Groin	Clavicular	Brow	Edge of symphysis pubis	St 30
Clavicular	Groin	Brow	Sternal end of clavicle	Ki 27
Shoulder	Navel	Throat	Tip of shoulder	LI 15
Navel	Shoulder	Throat	Next to umbilicus	Ki 16
Intercostal	Ear	Heart	Lateral aspect of ribs, sixth intercostal space	Sp 21
Ear	Intercostal	Heart	Base of ear	TH 17

When considering the role of the chakras in the treatment of musculo-skeletal conditions, it is sufficient to appreciate that they are very powerful acupuncture points and as such can be used in a variety of ways. Each of the seven major chakras has both a ventral and a spinal aspect, with the exception of the crown chakra, which is located at only one point on the top of the skull. The chakras and their levels are shown in Table 3.1.

The major chakras can become congested, over-stimulated or unco-ordinated. These imbalances can give rise to many symptoms within the physical body because each chakra is associated with one or two meridians, an endocrine gland, internal organs, spinal levels, autonomic nervous system and muscles, as well as having correspondences with the minor chakras. The associations are shown in Table 3.2.

It can be seen from Table 3.2 how extensive their influence is in the treatment of musculo-skeletal conditions. A book covering the whole of the chakra energy system is currently being prepared by the author.

Minor chakras

There are said to be 21 minor chakras, which are the reflected points of the majors. They consist of the spleen chakra and ten bilateral ones. For the purposes of this book, it is only necessary to mention the ten bilaterals; the spleen chakra has no musculo-skeletal relevance. However, the ten bilateral minor chakras are enormously important and, once learnt thoroughly, will become tried and tested friends that will be used time and time again. The minor chakras are each associated with a major chakra, as has been stated before, but also with another minor centre. The associations are shown in Table 3.3.

The minor chakras have particular influence in pain relief, especially in the peripheral joints and muscles. Techniques using this philosophy will be discussed fully later in the book.

4

Methods, techniques and sensations

Methods

The most common techniques of hands-on healing are performed with the tips and pads of the fingers and thumbs, with some use of the hands as a whole and occasionally of the ulnar border of the hands or even the elbow. There are six different ways of affecting the energy flow in an acupuncture point or a meridian/area:

1. Light touch on a point
2. Deep touch on a point
3. Gentle massage on a point
4. Stimulating massage on a point
5. Light massage on an area or meridian
6. Stimulating massage on an area or meridian.

A brief note here about cleanliness and hygiene. With all these techniques of acupressure, personal cleanliness and hygiene has to be exemplary. Fingernails *must* be trimmed short. Also, with the whole range of different techniques that the therapist will perform, the hands have to be very gentle as well as strong – so no rough skin. Please wear gloves when gardening and doing dirty work; always protect your hands and remember that they are your livelihood.

Light touch on a point

This is performed either with the forefinger or the middle finger pad, and is simply the placing of the finger on a point with hardly any pressure and with no other part of the hand in contact with the patient. The actual fingers that are used are very important, and this will be discussed at length later on.

Uses:

1. To transfer energy from a point or an area to another point or area. By touching various powerful acupoints and reflex points, the energic quality of internal organs or other areas of the body can be affected.
2. To draw away excess Yang (heat and inflammation) from a distal point or area.
3. To balance energy between two points. This can either be performed on two points of the same meridian to effect a natural flow of Ch'i or between a proximal point and a distal point of differing meridians. In the case of the latter, the distal point is called a great point.

Deep touch on a point

This technique can be performed with a single finger pad or with the fore-, middle or ring fingers in close proximity if there are adjacent acupoints to be treated. The fingers are placed on the acupoint or reflex point, very gently at first (always having regard for the patient's tissues, energy and aura) and progressively getting deeper and deeper into the tissues and working up to the patient's tolerance. This technique should *never* be painful or uncomfortable, and the pressure used should be tolerable and performed very slowly to accommodate the patient's pain threshold and comfort.

Uses:

1. In local inflammatory (Yang) areas, where the excess energy has to be dispersed either by placing just one finger on the area or by balancing that point with another point.
2. To release muscle spasm and tightness in the tissues and thus bring about harmony in the circulation (blood and lymphatics). Essentially, this technique of acupressure is for localized inflammatory areas where excess heat and inflammation need to be released. The therapist, with experience, may hold the point for up to 5 minutes whilst his or her fingers get progressively warmer. It is a technique that is very rewarding for the patient in the relief of pain. Like all the techniques shown, it is experience that will eventually lead to good results. The therapist must never be in a hurry to somehow force the movement of energy and thus establish a harmony. This will be stated over and over again in this book – never *will* things to happen; let them happen by themselves! Generally, it is the more chronic lesions that take longer to treat, as one would expect. The hold for this technique will last as long as pain or spasm persists or longer as the therapist sees fit – even when pain and spasm have eased, it is a comforting thing to carry on holding the point until total relaxation of the area has been achieved.

Gentle massage on a point

This is performed with the finger or thumb pads, and should be very gentle with no stimulation at all.

Uses:

1. To calm a patient, using certain acupressure/reflex points, prior to the main treatment. Such points as LI 4 and Li 3 come to mind here.
2. To treat sub-acute conditions where the underlying condition is chronic (Yin), but superficially it is essentially painful and inflamed (Yang).
3. In reflexology, this gentle form of massage may be performed on the feet and hand reflexes. Reflex points and many acupuncture points are reflected pathways of other points of subtle energy, and should not be 'blasted' with stimulating massage. Much more positive results will be obtained by using gentle massage than by digging the thumbs in and trying to bore a hole in the patient's tissues.

Gentle massage on a point should not be carried out in any condition where there is localized disease areas; e.g. growths, tumours, internal organ infection, rheumatoid joints etc. Disease can be likened to a force that can be easily spread (more about this in a later chapter). Conditions such as rheumatoid arthritis can be helped with acupressure, but never use stimulating massage. *Never, never, never* perform any stimulating massage in neurological conditions such as multiple sclerosis.

Stimulating massage on a point

This technique is very similar to circular friction as used in the treatment of soft tissue and sports injuries (how physiotherapists love these!). It is to be used *only* where there is a chronic or underlying chronic condition, and where energy needs to be created or stimulated. It can be performed with the ulnar border of the hand at the pisiform bone, or with the elbow when it is used on the spine. This is very popular in shiatsu.

Uses:

1. Treating localized chronic (Yin) conditions where the area needs stimulation of energy via the acupoints; for example, chronic tennis elbow or the local symptoms of frozen shoulder.
2. To stimulate the flow of energy down a meridian where there is chronic pain and discomfort at the distal end of the meridian; for example, massaging LI 4 for chronic sinusitis.
3. To stimulate the flow of lymphatic drainage by massaging the so-called neuro-lymphatic points or Chapman's reflexes. As previously mentioned, stimulating massage should not be performed on foot and hand reflexes (contrary to the popularly taught theories of zone therapy) in cases of neurological chronic disease. It is also contraindicated during the first 3 months of pregnancy and at menstruation.

Light massage on an area or meridian

This is performed with either the fingertips or the hand as a whole, and is simply the brushing of the skin with the gentlest of touches – *no*

stimulation whatsoever. Because of its subtlety there is no need to even touch the skin, and often the patient may keep the clothes on.
Uses:

1. On a meridian from the entry of the meridian to its exit – i.e. from the tsing point to the last point or *vice versa*, depending on whether energy in the meridian as a whole needs to be stimulated or sedated. Massage with the flow of energy to stimulate energy in the meridian, and against the flow of energy to sedate or lessen the energy flow.
2. When an area of the body is being prepared for more specific work at a later stage of treatment. This would constitute effleurage in orthodox massage.
3. In a diagnostic way when an area is palpated to ascertain certain underlying structural or soft tissue anomalies; for example, abdominal diagnosis.

Stimulating massage on an area or meridian

This is performed with a finger or thumb pad or with the inner border of the middle finger, and is essentially used as a stimulating massage in chronic illness.

It is used when a meridian or part of a meridian needs to be stimulated in order to bring more energy to the area or underlying organ connection. An example of this would be thumb-pad kneading along the course of the bladder meridian in chronic lumbar conditions. This technique of acupressure stimulates the stagnation of Ch'i energy due to a build-up of fatty deposits, scar tissue, fibrous tissue or cellulite. The whole length of the meridian need not be massaged, but as much as is practicable gives better results. This massage does not necessarily have to be performed with the flow of energy, but results will be improved if it is. Another example of using this technique is stimulating massage along the course of the large intestine and lung meridians in the treatment of chronic catarrh.

Connective tissue massage

There is one more type of stimulating massage that needs to be mentioned here; connective tissue massage. This may be performed along a meridian, around a joint or muscles, or on specified lines that are described when this wonderful form of massage is learnt thoroughly. The author first came into contact with it in 1973 when attending a course on the subject given by the late Maria Ebner FCSP DipTP. Being a qualified acupuncturist at the time, it was impressive to see the way that this form of massage could be used in energic depleted areas. A great debt is owed to this lady, who was one of the first to instil in her students the knowledge of the great power that therapists have in their hands and the importance of physical contact with patients. Although the theory of connective tissue massage (CTM) is not based on the oriental tradition of energy lines, it was found by experience that when the energy lines are stroked the results are better than when they are not, and that sometimes incredible pain relief in chronic conditions can be achieved when using it. There are courses run on this topic and books to be bought (e.g. Ebner, 1962), so it will not be described in detail here. CTM is performed with the radial border of the middle finger superimposed on the ring finger, and consists of three phases:

1. Contact with the patient to the required depth of the patient's tissues and at the correct starting point
2. Taking up the 'slack' of tissues by putting them on the stretch
3. A deep stroke, either short or long, along a prescribed line.

As those therapists with experience of CTM will know, there is sometimes a certain amount of unpleasant discomfort with this massage. If there is pain, the therapist must perform strokes across the meridian instead of long strokes. CTM is particularly helpful in chronic (Yin) conditions with sluggishness of circulation, lymph flow or the presence of scar tissue.

Sensations of acupressure

Having dealt with the various techniques and methods of using acupressure and discussed the types and uses, it seems appropriate at this juncture to consider the various sensations that the therapist feels under the fingers. The point is often made in this book that one of the great advantages of acupressure and its allied therapies is that the therapist can actually *feel* what is happening to the patient and may feel myriad different sensations. The following list is fairly comprehensive but certainly not exhaustive, for there are as many different sensations as there are practitioners performing these arts.

Heat

Probably the most common sensation that is felt under the finger pads is heat. This may occur for two reasons: first, it may be the patient's own heat that is felt; secondly, it may be heat that is being transferred to them by the therapist. Please note that *heat* transference and not energy (Ch'i) transference is emphasized here. As explained previously, no energy is imparted from the therapist to the patient; it is merely a question of using the patient's own healing energy in order to bring about homoeostasis and thus self-healing. Both of these give a slight hyperaemic effect, even with a very light touch. Heat may not be present straightaway and may take time to come through once the treatment has commenced, but when it does, try and hold the positions of the finger(s) for a few seconds in order to complete the balance and so create more harmony in the area. The patient may or may not feel a similar heat to you. Just because your patient does not feel any heat, it does not mean that the efficacy of the treatment is any less. Go by what is felt under the fingers, not necessarily by what the patient is feeling.

Pulsing

Another very common sensation is pulsing under the fingers. This happens especially when balancing two points, and is a signal an energy balance has been created that was not there before. As with heat, it may take a number of seconds to achieve and so patience is required. Initially the pulsing under the fingers may be erratic and irregular; the points need to be held gently until the pulsing is equal and regular. When this has been achieved, a balance of energy has been created between the two points. The more chronic the condition, the longer it will take to achieve the balance. If there are any obstructions such as fibrous or scar tissue around the area this may prevent easy balancing, but if patience is observed and rules are obeyed, balancing will happen. Patience is the key to most kinds of acupressure; it should not be rushed, and a balance of energy should never be willed or forced. Practice, though, makes perfect. Heat and pulsing may be present independently or together.

Tingling

There may also be tingling sensations present, and this is common when doing very subtle work. Sometimes the patient will experience a slight tingle or feeling of an electric shock (nothing unpleasant at all). Occasionally they will feel a real surge of energy that may affect them emotionally, and they may become quite tearful. This is often a good release of tension, and the patient will feel better for it. Be prepared and have a supply of paper tissues handy as well as a listening ear. It will be made clear later in the book how some seemingly musculo-skeletal conditions have emotional causes, and once these are released there is usually an outpouring of emotions before the physical condition improves (see Chapter 5). Other common releases of tension are yawning and sighing.

Cold and pain

Other less common sensations include feelings of cold or pain. Please do not confuse cold with being a negative sensation or emotion. It may or may not revert to being warm after a few seconds. Occasionally the patient may feel pain where none existed before. This is often caused by over-stimulation of the superficial *wei* energy (sensory and subcutaneous nerve endings) before the deeper balance of energy at the meridian level takes place. If the pain persists, gently move the hands slightly. If the pain persists more than a few seconds, then move on to another technique – it will be the patient's body telling the therapist that this is the wrong procedure.

Harmony

The other sensation that is often achieved is an overwhelming feeling of harmony and one-ness with the patient. Do not necessarily expect this every time. If the type and technique of acupressure is correct and the patient is attempting to balance him or herself energetically, then after a little while of holding the points a feeling of relaxation will follow for the patient as stress is released. The therapist's fingers or hands will seem to melt into the patient's tissues. The reasons for this are explained later in the chapter.

Types of acupressure

There are several types of clinical acupressure that can be used in the treatment of musculo-skeletal conditions. Those that are performed using the meridian system of energy are the use of local points, distal points, local and distal points, parallel points, great points, associated effect points, specific points and meridian massage. (The use of great points, associated effect points and specific points has been mentioned earlier.) There are other types of acupressure that do not make use of the meridians, and these are ear, temple, scalp, abdominal, hand and foot acupressure (the latter two more commonly called reflexology), and using the major and minor chakras.

Local points

These points are obviously local to the inflammatory or chronic part of the body that is being treated – for example, LI 11 in the treatment of tennis elbow or P 7 in the treatment of carpal tunnel syndrome. The technique and pressure that the therapist uses depends on the underlying condition and 'feel' of the tissues. In obvious acute conditions where there is heat, inflammation and some mild localized swelling, the therapist's finger(s) are gently placed on the points, *slowly* getting deeper and deeper into the tissues (to the patient's tolerance of discomfort) until there is obvious heat liberated in the area. There should be no massage as such, and the duration of treatment is very flexible and will depend on the amount of inflammation that needs to 'come out'. There is sometimes the need to hold a local point for up to 10 minutes. As with each and every operation, it is most important that the therapist tries not to will anything to happen or to hasten the healing process. Patients will respond at the rate they are meant to respond at, and each and every person is different! When there is an underlying sub-acute condition, albeit with a superficial inflammatory state, the fingers are placed as before and, when all the heat has been subdued, gentle circular massage is performed on the point in order to stimulate the underlying Yin condition. This is a very subtle art and has to be practised and practised in order to achieve perfection. In obvious chronic inflammatory conditions, such as chronic osteoarthritis, the local points are first gently stimulated with circular finger-pad massage, followed by more robust massage on the same point. In *all* chronic (Yin) conditions, energy needs to be summoned (stimulated) in order to be used! By using local points around a chronically arthritic joint over a period of several minutes, amazing pain relief and reduction of swelling can sometimes be achieved.

Distal points

This type of acupressure deals with affecting energy at a distance on a meridian that lies local to the condition but where localized treatment is impossible to do, such as with open wounds, conjunctivitis, rhinitis etc. The underlying meridian must be known, as treatment will be focussed either on the tsing (end) point or another point of great influence at the distal end of the meridian. Where the underlying condition is acute, the distant point should just be held until the heat and pain eases from the local area. Gentle massage should be used in sub-acute conditions and stimulating massage in chronic conditions when Ch'i energy has to be stimulated along the course of the meridian. Examples of using distal acupressure include the use of Bl 67 and St 45 in acute conjunctivitis, and the use of LI 4 and LI 1 in the treatment of acute toothache. Other types of distal acupressure use foot and hand reflexology, scalp reflexology, ear acupressure and points found in zonal acupressure. As stated previously, every part of the body has a number of associated (or reflected) points and areas, and there is usually a plethora of choice as to the treatment.

Local and distal points

The use of local and distal points together is the most common type of acupressure. So far this chapter has concentrated on single point acupressure; now there is a modality or attunement with clinical acupressure to consider, in that the therapist can actually feel what he or she is doing, including the pace of treatment. What is more, patients can often feel what is happening. After all, it is their energy system that is being affected. Patients who are used to acupressure treatment will often tell the therapist that a change in sensation has taken place before the therapist feels it. The various sensations that therapists may feel have already been described, and the essential thing that has to be remembered with this type of acupressure is that therapists are *balancing* energy between two points – nothing more, nothing less. They are *not* imparting any of their energy or taking part in any mystical 'healing'. There are several ways of performing local and distal point acupressure:

1. Balancing points that are on the same meridian
2. Balancing points using the local point and a great point that is not on the same meridian as the distal point
3. Balancing points using the local point and a major reflex point (foot, hand, ear, scalp)
4. Balancing points using the local point and the nearest chakra point
5. Balancing points that lie on the same zone of energy
6. Balancing points using the local point and its parallel point.

The anatomy of reflexes, chakras and zones was discussed in Chapter 3, and the rationale is the same as balancing energy using local and distal points on the same meridian.

Example of balancing points on the same meridian – occipital headache

The points used are GB 20 and GB 41. The therapist places the middle finger of either hand on point GB 20 nearest the site of pain of the occipital headache and touches gently for a few seconds so that the patient gets used to the feel. The middle finger of the other hand is then introduced on to GB 41 and the therapist holds the two points, sitting comfortably, until the pulsing or heat appears under the fingers as explained earlier. The patient should find that the pain has either gone or changed after a couple of minutes. It is possible to move the pain, and the therapist has to be prepared for this and be ready go on to another set of points if necessary. The balance of energy has been achieved when the sensation under both fingers is the same. Where the occipital pain is chronic the distal point may have to be stimulated slightly, but not too much!

Example of balancing points using a great point – occipital headache

'Great points' are those acupoints on the body that have more energy influence and are used for more than one purpose, as explained in Chapter 2. Occipital headache is purposely used again as an example in order to illustrate how the same condition may be treated using two different approaches. This is also a way of stressing that there are no hard and fast rules when it comes to acupressure healing. The points used are GB 20 and LI 4. As discussed earlier, LI 4 is an extremely important point that is used for painful conditions around the face, head and upper chest. The same procedure is carried out as before, with the slight exception that LI 4 will need more gentle stimulation than a point that is on the same meridian. The therapist will note that, when using these points, a balance of energy will be effected quite quickly, but this does not necessarily immediately help the pain. The reason for this is that pain is a complex issue and has come about because of the patient's complex physiological changes; therefore it is not always possible to ease deep-seated pain immediately. What the therapist can do, however, is hold the points for much longer than needed merely to attain a balance of energy. The longer the points are held, the better and more long-lasting will be the results. It is very helpful to hold the points until a shift of energy or a change of emphasis occurs. This sensation is dealt with later in this chapter.

Parallel points

Parallel point acupressure is the use of the same point on the opposite limb. It is used when it is impossible to do local point acupressure, e.g. gravitational ulcer, or it can be used as an adjunct to other forms of acupressure. It seems to be highly effective in certain conditions.

When there is discontinuity of the skin (ulceration) or a burn etc. and it is therefore impossible to place ones fingers locally, the *exact* point on the opposite limb is used. Taking the example of a gravitational ulcer, which occurs around the lower two-thirds of the medial aspect of the tibia and is quite often centred on point Sp 6, the treatment is to stimulate the opposite Sp 6 for anything up to 5 minutes. Other points can also be stimulated as long as they are parallel to the acute or chronic inflammation. They do not necessarily have to be meridian points, but if they are on a meridian it will enhance the treatment.

Parallel point acupressure can also be performed as an adjunct to other types of acupressure. For instance, in the case of a very painful medial aspect of the knee, as well as performing local and distal acupressure and balancing 'through' the lesion along the kidney meridian, the painful point on the knee can be balanced with the *exact* same point on the other knee. Once again the points are held until a balance of energy is felt under the fingers, but it is often a good idea to keep the hold on for up to 5 minutes. Some amazing results can be obtained with this procedure.

Meridian massage

Meridian massage can be used for both stimulation and sedation.

Stimulation

This is performed either with finger pad or thumb pad kneading along the meridian, and is done in the direction of energy flow (i.e. from the tsing point to the end point). This stimulates energy flow and is useful in underlying chronic conditions; for example, thumb-pad kneading along the course of the bladder and kidney meridians would be given in all cases of osteoarthritis. It is a very helpful technique with which to commence treatment, and eases stagnation of Ch'i along the course of the channel due to fatty deposits, cellulite or fibrositic nodules. The whole length of the meridian need not necessarily be massaged if the condition is purely a local one, but the more of the meridian that can be massaged, the better will be the results.

A stimulating type of massage can also be performed, using the whole hand and brushing along the meridian in the direction of energy flow. It can even be performed through thin clothing, and can be quite effective in the initial stimulation of energy in the particular meridian that is being treated.

Sedation

Using a light touch, either with the fingertips or the whole hand, the meridian is massaged in the opposite direction to the energy flow (i.e. from the end point to the tsing point). The result is that excess energy is removed from the area or from the underlying cause. It is extremely influential where there is acute pain, spasm, heat and inflammation in the area – for example, light touch massage along the course of the the gall bladder meridian will help in acute tendonitis, wherever it happens to be. Several strokes along the meridian can be carried out and, again, it is most useful if performed at the commencement of the treatment.

The physiology of sensations felt in acupressure

The paradigm that is called acupressure falls under the umbrella of what is generally termed 'energy medicine'. Mention has been made earlier of this energy and what various philosophers and cultures down the ages have called it – names ranging from medicatrix naturae and Ch'i to Prana and Odic force (see Chapter 1). Before the advent of scientific medicine, it was impossible to quantify this healing energy in any way – people who 'healed' simply knew of its existence. Today, most people in the 'healing' professions tend to call it vital or life force. In the later stages of the twentieth century we are a little more enlightened as to what vital force actually is and what happens between healer and patient during a hands-on (or hands-off) treatment.

Rhythyms and cycles

It can be said that life on this planet is controlled, nourished and maintained by various cycles and rhythms. There are the naturally occurring cycles of the seasons, the lunar cycle and the solar cycle. The lunar cycle alone has incredible ramifications on life on the planet – the gravitational magnetic influence of the moon has the power to move the oceans of the world, and indeed to move water within each and every one of us. We tend to gain weight during the few days around full moon, and there have been scores of experiments performed, in laboratory conditions, that show how even the humble potato gains weight during the phase of the full moon. Women have a menstrual cycle that varies from 18–40 days, and we are all subject to the three circadian life cycles of 24, 31 and 35 days duration. This knowledge is used in the science of biofeedback. In traditional Chinese and Japanese medicine it is said that humans are subject to various energy patterns in their bodies over a 24-hour period. Each of the 12 main organs has a peak of energy over a 2-hour period. It is found in practice that certain acupuncture points are more 'open' at particular times of the day, month and season. This is a branch of traditional medicine called celestial stems.

Research has been carried out into the frequencies that appear in the aura and whether or not the frequency changes around the powerful acupuncture and reflex points on the body, especially the chakras, are different to those at non-acupuncture parts of the body. Dr Valerie Hunt, a psychologist and biophysicist, has successfully analysed frequency patterns that correlate with known illnesses, states of mental activity and healing mindset frequencies, and has found a consistent correlation between recorded frequencies and reported auric colours and other vibrational patterns 'seen' by psychics and clairvoyants. The working hypotheses derived from this research are that all living systems generate a bio-energy field or aura that acts as an expression of the vital force, that the mind has field properties, and that the frequency-banded aura interacts with the auras of other living systems and with geomagnetic and subtle energy field of the chakras (Hunt, 1995).

The late Maxwell Cade studied medicine and psychology at London University and then specialized in radio-navigation and radiation physics. He founded a biofeedback laboratory in London during the 1960s and 1970s and pioneered bi-hemisphere EEG recordings and combined frequency and voltage amplitude profiles, using equipment called the 'Mind Mirror'. He tested hundreds of healers, patients receiving healing, yogis, meditators and 'ordinary' people, correlating profiles that he found were typical of different states of awareness through a nine-stage hierarchy of deep sleep, dreaming sleep, hypnogogic, waking, meditative and healing, lucid awareness, creativity, 'God' consciousness or illumination, to 'cosmic' consciousness. The working hypothesis is that, when both cerebral hemispheres are resonating at around 7–8 Hz (low alpha, high amplitude) and the mind is in a transcendental meditation (TM) or intention-to-heal mindset or higher state, we enter into a state of consciousness that transcends physical boundaries and can interact with others.

From the above, it seems that 'healing' takes place when the brain wave rhythm of the patient is about 7–8 Hz, and that this is augmented when the practitioner or healer has the same rhythm as the patient. This explains the 'one-ness' that was mentioned earlier in this chapter.

The five states of brainwave frequencies are as follows:

1. Beta rhythm – 13–30 Hz. This is the normal waking rhythm of the brain associated with active thinking, focussing on the outside world and solving problems. Anxiety states and muscular activity send the frequency into the upper ranges of 30 Hz plus.
2. Alpha rhythm – 8–13 Hz. Alpha is the most prominent rhythm in the whole realm of brain activity. It denotes an empty mind rather than a relaxed one, a mindless state rather than a passive one. This is the state known as daydreaming. It happens frequently during the day, even driving a car, when a driver can cover miles of familiar roads without the total concentration of beta rhythm. Also in this mind set is the 'other worldly' sensation when outside influences are cut off and one becomes oblivious to the surroundings (very good when writing books!!!)
3. Alpha/theta rhythm – around 8 Hz. This is the rhythm where there is said to be energy transfer and a one-ness with the patient/client. Both the healer and patient are in a state of relaxation. In practical terms in acupressure, the sensation is quite marked (even taking into account the subtlety of what is happening). There appears to be a 'shift' of sensation under the fingers; this is usually a lovely gentle warmth where none was before. Often, though not always, the patient feels the shift at the same time. This begins the time of one-ness between the therapist and the patient, and it is essential that this state of awareness is reached, especially when treating chronic conditions, before healing takes place. The phrase 'a shift of energy emphasis' will be repeated several times in this book. This is where the therapist and the patient attune together at 8 Hz.
4. Theta rhythm – 4–7 Hz. This frequency appears in dreaming or in the half-awake hypnogogic state with dreamlike imagery. Theta appears as consciousness slips towards drowsiness.

5. Delta rhythm – 1/2–4 Hz. This is primarily associated with deep sleep. There have also been reports that delta waves appear at the onset of paranormal phenomena, and that they are also associated with the higher levels of consciousness.

5

Relationships and associations

This chapter is dedicated to the myriad different relationships that exist within the human body that the therapist will need to know in order to use acupressure as a total treatment regimen. Mention has been made in earlier chapters of some of the various relationships, such as parallel points and zones, but this chapter will focus on the several relationships that exist with the spine, muscles and all the peripheral joints. Mention will also be made of 'listening posts'.

Relationships of the spine

Lovett brother

The old song goes: 'the footbone is connected to the heel bone, the heel bone is connected to the leg bone ...' and so on. Therapists often forget this very simple fact – that with every trauma and subsequent lesion, unless that lesion is treated correctly within a few days, there will be a resultant lesion elsewhere in the musculo-skeletal structure. For example, a misplaced atlas bone that is causing headaches and migraine may have become malaligned due not to direct trauma, such as a whiplash injury, but to an earlier trauma to the base of the spine or even the ankle. Therefore, in manipulative therapy of any type it is pointless simply to adjust the offending vertebra without making sure that the other vertebrae are correctly positioned. In other words, the *cause* of the lesion has to be treated; if it is not, the same symptoms will recur.

The upper and lower spine function in a synchronous manner. As the atlas rotates right, the fifth lumbar rotates right – thus, the fifth lumbar vertebra is the Lovett brother of the atlas. The same synchronization is true of the axis with the fourth lumbar vertebra, and the third cervical with the third lumbar vertebra. From that point there is a shift, and the fourth cervical vertebra goes the opposite way to the

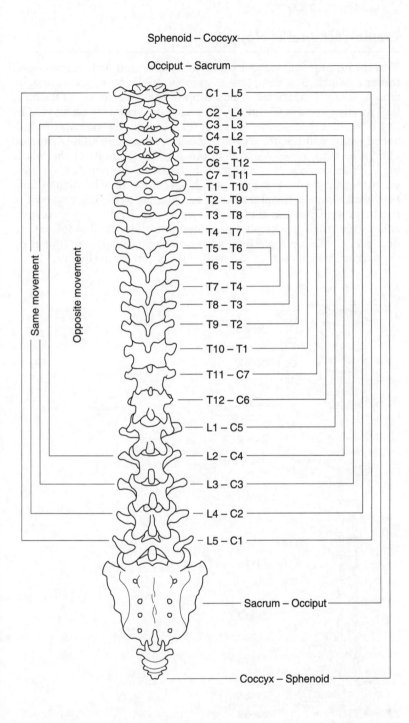

Sphenoid – Coccyx

Occiput – Sacrum

C1 – L5
C2 – L4
C3 – L3
C4 – L2
C5 – L1
C6 – T12
C7 – T11
T1 – T10
T2 – T9
T3 – T8
T4 – T7
T5 – T6
T6 – T5
T7 – T4
T8 – T3
T9 – T2
T10 – T1
T11 – C7
T12 – C6
L1 – C5
L2 – C4
L3 – C3
L4 – C2
L5 – C1

Sacrum – Occiput

Coccyx – Sphenoid

Same movement

Opposite movement

Figure 5.1 The spine, showing Lovett brothers.

second lumbar vertebra, etc., until the upper and lower spine meet at the fifth and sixth thoracic vertebrae (Figure 5.1). This knowledge is vital to the therapist in order to be able to balance the energies between the upper and the lower spine. When there is an obvious lesion anywhere in the spine, as well as balancing all the necessary points (see Chapter 8), the Lovett brother must also be balanced.

Cranio-sacral reflexology

This useful practical subject is not to be confused with cranio-sacral therapy, which is a complete system of medicine in its own right. Cranio-sacral reflexology is based upon the 'five zones' philosophy that was discussed in Chapter 3. To recap, the body may be divided by five bilateral vertical zones and painful areas on one zone may be balanced using acupressure with the tender reflex point that is situated along the same zone. As well as the vertical divisions of the whole body, there are also vertical (and horizontal) divisions within each section of the body. For example, the great toe may be divided into five vertical and horizontal zones, each relating to the relevant part of the head and also the thumb! In cranio-sacral reflexology, vertical zones exist from the occipital protuberance of the skull to the superior aspect of the sacrum. There are also imaginary horizontal lines on the sacrum, which correspond with various vertebrae (Figure 5.2).

Figure 5.2   Spinal and sacral zones in cranio-sacral reflexology.

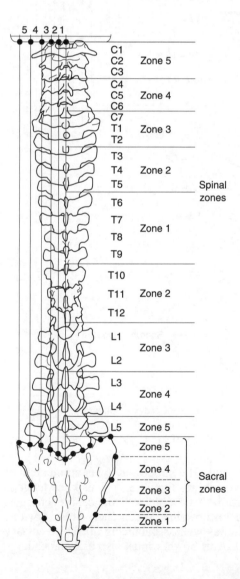

In practical terms there are several ways that we can use this knowledge, in both diagnosis and treatment. The following represent some examples:

1. A tender point on gentle palpation of the nuchal line along the occipital protuberance will tell the therapist not only that there may be underlying localized inflammation, but also that the corresponding vertebrae will need treatment.
2. Tender points on gentle palpation along the superior border of the sacrum may not just indicate sacral pain, but also that the associated vertebra needs treatment. Whenever there is tenderness on a certain point at either the occiput or the sacrum, there will *always* be a reciprocal tenderness in the other one on the same vertical zone. These two may be energically balanced using gentle pressure on both points until there is unison of sensation. When this happens, it means that the energy line that lies between the two is balanced and that the vertebra concerned should also be eased. The reader can immediately see that this represents an excellent initial procedure in the treatment of any spinal condition.
3. Tenderness on gentle palpation along the outer borders (left and right) of the sacrum indicates imbalance with a corresponding vertebra as well as imbalance along the associated generalized zone in the body. This may also indicate various imbalances occurring at an organic level, such as those organs concerned with circulation, respiration, digestion, glandular functions and elimination.
4. Tenderness on gentle palpation along any of the paravertebral vertical zones obviously indicates imbalance in the underlying tissues (pain, spasm, induration of circulation or lymph etc.), but may also indicate underlying organic changes, muscle imbalance or imbalance at either the occiput or the sacrum.

If this philosophy seems hard to accept, please, please remember that the body represents a marvellous web of interconnected reflexes, each with its own way of showing the practitioner the true cause of the particular condition. Therefore, if tender points are felt on the nuchal line, or on the superior or lateral aspects of the sacrum, note should be taken to which zone it belongs because this indicates that there is some kind of imbalance in the related horizontal zone(s) on the spine. This, of course, could mean any one of a score of different musculoskeletal conditions, but by doing this the therapist is 'clearing the wood to get to the trees' and localizing where the imbalance lies. This makes life much simpler, and enables some diagnostic shortcuts to be taken.

Effects of spinal misalignments

This short section is common knowledge to any therapist who has undertaken a long manipulative course, and is taken as biblical truth by the majority of osteopathic and chiropractic colleges. Figure 5.3 represents a diagram taken from a book on applied kinesiology, which is a modern offshoot of chiropractic (Walther, 1976). It shows the effect of spinal misalignments, often called 'subluxations' or 'fixations'

Chart of effects of Spinal Misalignments

Every area of the body is controlled by nerves. The normal function of these nerves can be disturbed by misalignments of the vertebrae affecting the disease conditions shown below.

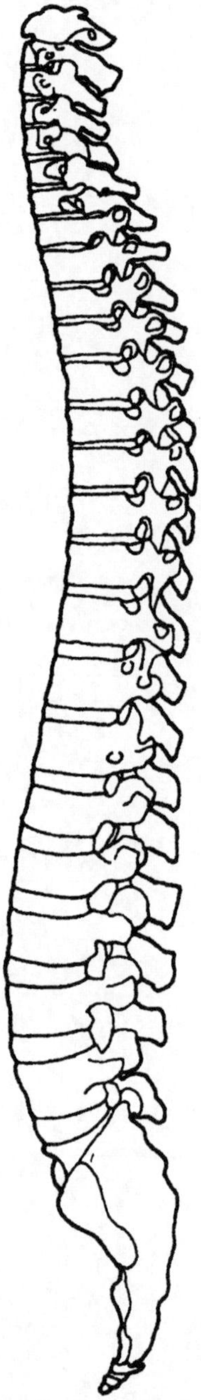

Vertebrae	Areas	Effects
1C	Blood supply to the head, the pituitary gland, the scalp, bones of the face, the brain itself, inner and middle ear, the sympathetic nervous system.	Headaches, nervousness, insomnia, head colds, high blood pressure, migraine headaches, mental conditions, nervous breakdowns, amnesia, sleeping sickness, chronic tiredness, dizziness or vertigo, St. Vitus dance.
2C	Eyes, optic nerve, auditory nerve, sinuses, mastoid bones, tongue and forehead.	Sinus trouble, allergies, crossed eyes, deafness, erysipelas, eye trouble, earache, fainting spells, certain cases of blindness.
3C	Cheeks, outer ear, face bones, teeth, trifacial nerve.	Neuralgia, acne or pimples, eczema.
4C	Nose, lips, mouth, eustachian tube.	Hay fever, catarrh, hard of hearing, adenoids.
5C	Vocal cords, neck glands, pharynx.	Laryngitis, hoarseness, throat conditions like a sore throat or quinsy.
6C	Neck muscles, shoulders, tonsils.	Stiff neck, pain in upper arm, tonsillitis, whooping cough, croup.
7C	Thyroid gland, bursae in the shoulder, the elbows.	Bursitis, colds, thyroid conditions.
1T	Arms from the elbow down, including the hands, wrists and fingers, also the oesophagus and trachea.	Asthma, cough, difficult breathing, shortness of breath, pain in lower arms and hand.
2T	Heart including its valves and covering, also coronary arteries.	Functional heart conditions and certain chest pains.
3T	Lungs, bronchial tubes, pleura, chest, breast, nipples.	Bronchitis, pleurisy, pneumonia, congestion, influenza.
4T	Gall bladder and common duct.	Gall bladder conditions, jaundice, shingles.
5T	Liver, solar plexus, blood.	Liver conditions, fevers, low blood pressure, anaemia, poor circulation, arthritis.
6T	Stomach.	Stomach troubles including nervous stomach, indigestion, heartburn, dyspepsia.
7T	Pancreas, islands of Langerhans, duodenum.	Diabetes, ulcers, gastritis.
8T	Spleen, diaphragm	Hiccoughs, lowered resistance.
9T	Adrenals or supra-renals.	Allergies, hives.
10T	Kidneys.	Kidney troubles, hardening of the arteries, chronic tiredness, nephritis, pyelitis.
11T	Kidneys, ureters.	Skin conditions like acne, pimples, eczema, or boils.
12T	Small intestines, fallopian tubes, lymph circulation.	Rheumatism, gas pains, certain types of sterility.
1L	Large intestines or colon, inguinal rings.	Constipation, colitis, dysentery, diarrhoea, rupturing or hernias.
2L	Appendix, abdomen, upper leg, caecum	Appendicitis, cramps, difficult breathing, acidosis varicose veins.
3L	Sex organs, ovaries or testicles, uterus, bladder, knee.	Bladder troubles, menstrual troubles, like painful or irregular periods, miscarriages, bed wetting, impotency, change of life symptoms, many knee pains.
4L	Prostrate gland, muscles of the lower back, sciatic nerve.	Sciatica, lumbago, difficult, painful, or too frequent urination, backaches.
5L	Lower legs, ankles, feet, toes, arches.	Poor circulation in the legs, swollen ankles, weak ankles and arches, cold feet, weakness in the legs, leg cramps.
Sacrum	Hip bones, buttocks.	Sacro-iliac conditions, spinal curvatures.
Coccyx	Rectum, anus.	Haemorrhoids or piles, pruritis, itching, pain at end of spine on sitting.

Figure 5.3   Chart of effects of spinal misalignments. Adapted from Thie, J. F. (1979). *Touch for Health – A New Approach to Restoring Our Natural Energies*, DeVorss and Co.

by chiropractors. Whenever there is a misalignment, nervous tissue is stretched around the lesion. This nerve tissue could be motor or sensory, but is often sympathetic or parasympathetic in origin. It is often the autonomic nerve anomalies that cause the various effects of each individual vertebral misalignment. It is most helpful for the therapist to be aware of this philosophy but, as each and every human is a unique individual, it can only be used as a guide. Please note that this is quite different to the back transporting points or the associated effect points of traditional Chinese medicine that were discussed in Chapter 3; these represent the imbalance to the internal organs and subsequent symptoms due to the energic, whereas Figure 5.3 represents imbalance due to nerve deviation. However, each is as valid as the other.

Relationships of muscles

Neuro-lymphatic massage points – Chapman's reflexes

Dr Frank Chapman, an osteopath, discovered the 'Chapman's reflexes' in the 1930s. He found that by stimulating a specific point, it would increase lymphatic drainage in a specific organ. The locations of these reflexes are primarily along the anterior intercostal spaces down to the pubis, and posteriorly along the spine (Figure 5.4). Some reflexes are located in the legs and arms. Active reflexes can usually be palpated, and are quite tender in the anterior of the body. The tenderness is usually in direct ratio to the chronicity and severity of the condition. The reflexes on the anterior of the body are small and located in the subcutaneous fat, and often feel like a small pea or bean. The posterior ones are usually less tender and more difficult to palpate; the feeling here is more diffuse and less specific. Treatment of the neuro-lymphatic reflex (NL) is done with the finger pads in a rotatory manner. The reflex will need a very firm pressure, especially in chronic conditions – it is hardly a subtle treatment, and is in fact one of the most painful procedures that can be done in the whole field of 'bodywork'. The good news, though, is that it works! Chapman's reflexes, which were used for three decades in order to improve generalized lymphatic obstruction, went through a transformation in the 1960s, when George Goodheart correlated all of them with specific muscle associations. It has been found by subsequent eminent chiropractors and professionals, using applied kinesiology, that deep massage on the NL reflex can produce an immediate freeing of congestion in the associated muscle, especially in chronic imbalance, and subsequently help to strengthen it. Although this is not strictly acupressure, it represents a very useful adjunct in the treatment of musculo-skeletal conditions.

There are two ways in which neuro-lymphatic massage may be used; either by massaging the points directly associated with the muscle that needs strengthening, for example massage along the underside of the costal angle to affect the quadriceps, or by giving a full body massage. The latter is by far the more beneficial; although some

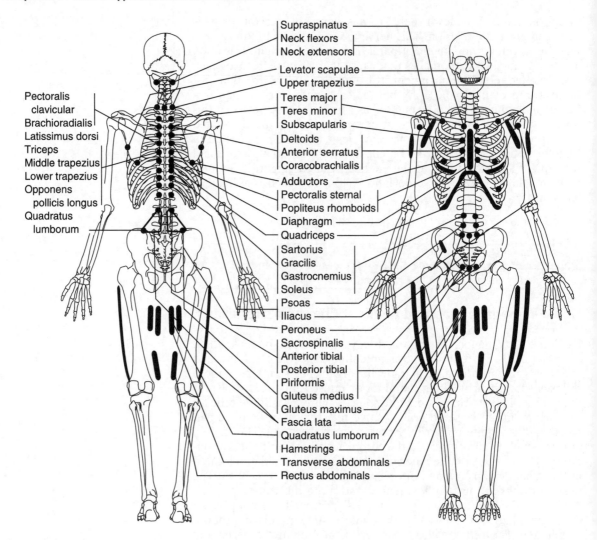

Figure 5.4 Neuro-lymphatic massage points.

points may be painful the whole procedure only takes about 1 minute with practice, and it is a wonderful way of making sure that the lymphatic stagnation that occurs in chronic muscular imbalance is freed prior to the main thrust of the treatment. The patient must be warned that it may be a painful procedure. The areas that are most painful are on the ilio-tibial tract and tensor fascia latae. These unfortunately need to be treated in all cases of chronic low back pain. In the case of specific acute muscular conditions, it is only necessary to massage the NL of the individual muscle.

Organic and meridian associations

Physical therapists are used to dealing with muscular spasms that occur around a lesion as a self-healing mechanism of protection. Often they are taught to massage the spasm in order to 'soften up' the muscle, hence allowing adequate flow of blood, lymph (and Ch'i) to the muscle and the underlying soft tissues and thus being able to align

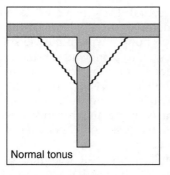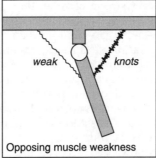

weak   knots

Normal tonus   Opposing muscle weakness

Figure 5.5 Normal tonus and opposing muscle weakness.

joints that have been pulled out of alignment due to spasm. This was the cornerstone of the treatment of muscular imbalance by physical therapists, osteopaths and chiropractors until the early 1960s. It was then that George Goodheart came up with a new idea for working with muscles. Goodheart concluded that it wasn't really muscle spasm that caused pain and vertebral misalignment, but that weak muscles on one side of the body can cause normal muscles opposing to become or seem tight. When a tight or knotted muscle is found, the first reaction is, as before, to work directly on the muscle itself. If, however the underlying joint misalignment has not been rectified, the tension, even if temporarily released, will return. Think of a door held in place by two springs, so that it can swing either way (Figure 5.5). As long as the tension on both springs is equal, the system will be in balance. If, however, one spring weakens, the opposing spring ties itself in knots taking up the slack. No amount of oiling the knotted spring will rebalance the system; the weak spring has to be strengthened.

Goodheart's research showed that most muscles have an association with internal organs via the meridian system. He devised a system of therapy called applied kinesiology, which is an offshoot of chiropractic. Applied kinesiology (AK) states that muscles can be tested

Table 5.1 The associations of organs, meridians and muscles

Organ/meridian	*Muscle*
Conception	Supraspinatus
Governor	Teres major
Stomach	Pectoralis major (clavicular), levator scapula, neck flexors and extensors, biceps, brachioradialis
Spleen	Latissimus dorsi, trapezius (middle and lower fibres), opponens pollicis longus, triceps
Heart	Subscapularis
Small intestine	Quadriceps, abdominals (all)
Bladder	Peroneus, sacrospinalis (all), anterior tibials, posterior tibials
Kidney	Psoas major/iliacus, trapezius (upper fibres)
Pericardium	Gluteus medius, adductors (all), piriformis, gluteus maximus
Triple heater	Teres minor, sartorius, gracilis, soleus, gastrocnemius
Gall bladder	Deltoid (anterior fibres), popliteus
Liver	Pectoralis major (sternal part), rhomboids
Lung	Serratus anterior, coracobrachialis, deltoid, diaphragm
Large intestine	Tensor fascia latae, hamstrings

to see how strong or weak they are, and that it is the weak muscles that need to be strengthened in order to create a balance of energy in the muscle, organ and meridian. It is not the type of muscle strength testing that physical therapists are used to doing and it is not a question of brute force; rather it is a method of using very subtle holding techniques to see if the muscle spindle contracts or 'takes'. The association of each organ, meridian and muscle is shown in Table 5.1. This in no way covers every muscle in the body, but the therapist should be able to utilize this knowledge in the treatment of 99 per cent of musculo-skeletal conditions.

This knowledge has profound implications in the treatment of musculo-skeletal conditions. Very many conditions that seem to be of a mechanical nature may *not* have a mechanical aetiology. They may be caused by organic, Ch'i, lymphatic or emotional conditions, and the seemingly mechanical condition is merely where the patient is housing the symptoms. It is therefore not always in the best interest of the patient just to treat the symptoms without ascertaining the root cause. A very good way of ascertaining if the cause is a mechanical one is to ask the patient how the condition first happened. If the answer is that it was a direct injury, sprain, blow or trauma, then the local symptoms may be treated with any of the physiotherapeutic methods that have been tried and tested over the years. If the answer to the question is that 'it just happened' or 'it crept up slowly', then we are not dealing with mechanical aetiology and the therapist has to find out what the real cause is. Of course the local symptoms have to be eased, in order to help the patient, but unless the cause is located and balanced energically, the symptoms will return!!

Acupressure holding points

This section naturally leads on from the previous one. The science of applied kinesiology, which has been with the profession since the early 1960s, gave rise to something called 'touch for health', which could be described as a way of testing and balancing muscle energy that anyone, even lay people, can use. Touch for health was brought to the UK in the early 1970s by Brian Butler. It is now extremely popular and is taught by several colleges, each using different slants and approaches. One of the universal techniques taught by every college is the acupressure holding points, which can be used to strengthen or weaken a given muscle. It has already been stated that each muscle is associated with a particular energy channel (meridian) and that if the muscle becomes weakened through trauma, it can be energically balanced by using the acupressure holding points. For each muscle there are four points to be learnt; two points are balanced, followed by another two. The exact points that are used are based upon the law of five elements (see Chapter 1), using the accumulation points of the Sheng or the Ko cycles. The first two points are held for about 30 seconds, or until a warmth and unity is felt under the fingers; this is followed by holding the second two points for an equal length of time. With most acupressure it will be more common to stimulate or strengthen the muscles; only occasionally will it be necessary to sedate or weaken a muscle. The exception is when all else has been tried to ease the spasm in a particular area. It is most important *never* to sedate the heart meridian when working with the subscapularis muscle (the only muscle associated with the heart meridian); rather, the couple of the heart meridian, namely the small intestine meridian, should be stimulated. Figure 5.6 shows the stimulation and sedation points for the meridians and subsequent muscles.

Relationship of muscles, organs, meridians, vertebrae and major and minor chakras

The previous section dealt with the various muscle associations with meridians/organs. Later research by applied kinesiologists has narrowed the field of muscle associations to specific organs that may or may not be the same as the associated meridian. This represents another leap forward in our understanding of the many energic associations that exist within the human frame. The author's own research over the past 15 years has taken this work forward two stages. First, there is now a vertebral level associated with each muscle. This is where the therapist touches to create an energy balance with the muscle involved. The exact point of contact is in the space below the spinous process of the vertebra. Please do not confuse the associated vertebra with the many and various nerve connections to a muscle originating in the spine – attempting to rationalize any neural connection will only confuse. These relationships have been worked out as a result of years of research, and represent the energy flow from one to another. Secondly, there is another of the author's 'pet' subjects, namely the major and minor chakras (these were outlined in Chapter 3). In the treatment of musculo-skeletal conditions, they represent powerful acupuncture points that have been found, in practice, to be better than the standard acupuncture points of pain relief etc. in respect of results obtained. This statement is purely subjective – the claims made are as a result of years of research and trial and error on unsuspecting but gratified patients! The reader will note that each and every muscle has a different 'formula' of relationships, thus making each muscular balance unique to that muscle. Please note that there is no need to distinguish between sedation and stimulation of the energy flow to a muscle. By using this technique the muscle energy is balanced; where weak before it becomes strong, and where in spasm before, it becomes normal. It does not mean that this technique represents a one-off instant miracle of bodywork. As well as doing the acupressure balancing, the therapist should follow the other procedures of massage, mobilizing and relaxation techniques.

The method involved is as follows:

1. The muscle to be balanced is identified, either by the pain, spasm or congestion it has, or because on testing the strength of the muscle it has been shown to be weak. Also, because the therapist already knows the associated organs, if the organ is showing signs of distress the associated muscle will always be in a state of imbalance. Therefore, as well as providing homoeostasis in the muscle concerned, the energy quality of the organ is also enhanced.

Stimulation   Sedation

Lung

Serratus anterior
Deltoid
Diaphragm
Coracobrachialis

Large intestine

Tensor fascia l.
Hamstrings
Quadratus
lumborum

Stomach

Pectoralis major
(Clavicular head)
Levator scapula
Neck flexors
Neck extensors
Biceps
Brachioradialis

Figure 5.6   a. Stimulation and sedation points: lung, large intestine and stomach.

2.   The associated meridian is stroked in the direction of the energy flow if the muscle needs to be strengthened. It is very unusual that massage along the meridian for this purpose needs to be performed in the opposite way.

3.   The relevant vertebral level is found and held by the pad of (usually) the middle finger. In the case of multiple vertebral levels, as in the case of the abdominals and the sacrospinalis, each

Stimulation   Sedation

Spleen

Latissimus dorsi
Trapezius (lower
and middle fibres)
Opponens pollicis
Triceps
Extensor digitorum

Heart

Subscapularis

Small intestine

Quadriceps
Abdominals (all)

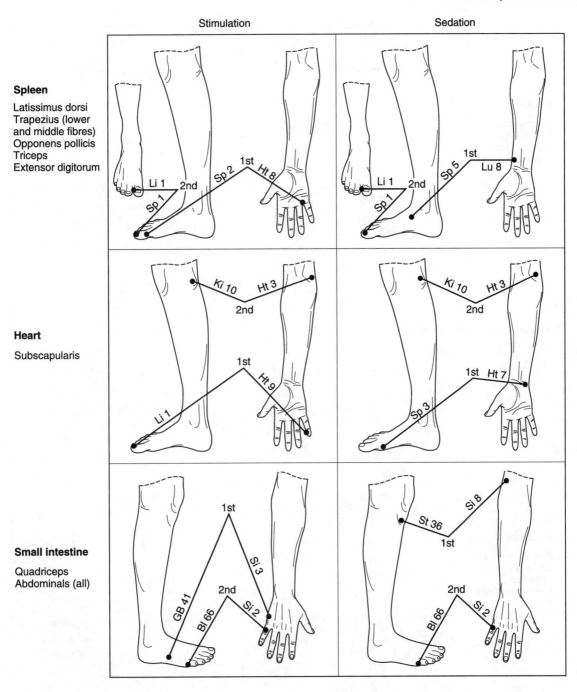

level must be balanced in turn. The middle finger of the other hand is then placed on the relevant major chakra point (frontal point) and a balance of energy achieved as described previously; this may take a couple of minutes, although often just 30 seconds.

3.   A finger is kept on the spinal point and is now balanced with the relevant minor chakra point, this is invariably a point on the

Figure 5.6 b. Stimulation and sedation points: spleen, heart and small intestine.

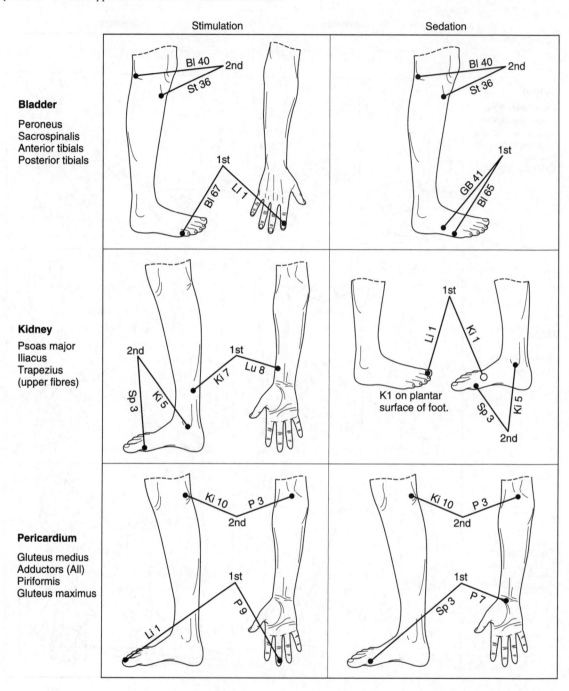

Stimulation   Sedation

Bladder

Peroneus
Sacrospinalis
Anterior tibials
Posterior tibials

Kidney

Psoas major
Iliacus
Trapezius
(upper fibres)

K1 on plantar
surface of foot.

Pericardium

Gluteus medius
Adductors (All)
Piriformis
Gluteus maximus

Figure 5.6 c. Stimulation and sedation points: bladder, kidney and pericardium.

periphery of the body and quite easy to find. This balance should take another 30 seconds to a minute.

4.   Finally the points of the major and minor chakra points need to be balanced with each other. This should take very little time. The muscle is then in a much more relaxed state so that either the therapist is able treat the underlying joint condition with further acupressure treatment or the muscle that surrounds or supports a

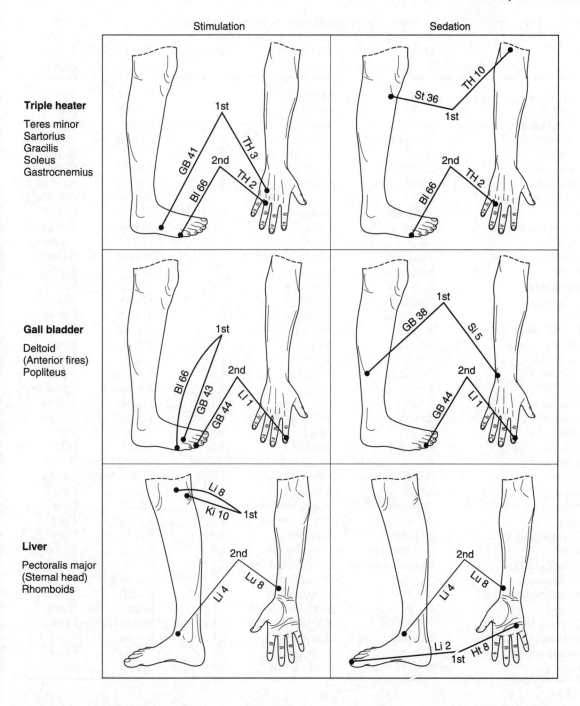

Triple heater

Teres minor
Sartorius
Gracilis
Soleus
Gastrocnemius

Gall bladder

Deltoid
(Anterior fires)
Popliteus

Liver

Pectoralis major
(Sternal head)
Rhomboids

Figure 5.6 d. Stimulation and sedation points: triple heater, gall bladder and liver.

weakened joint is stronger. Table 5.2 shows the various associations discussed.

Table 5.2 may, at first glance, seem to be slightly daunting. There are a couple of ways of making it easier to remember. First, it is imperative that the practitioner knows body anatomy, otherwise he or she will be lost completely. The origins and insertions of each muscle

Table 5.2   Associations of the muscles, organs, meridians, vetebrae and chakras

Muscle	Organ	Meridian	Vertebra	Major chakra	Minor chakra
Sternomastoid	Sinus	Stomach	C1	Crown	Ear
Facial muscles	Sinus	Governor	C1–2	Crown	Ear
Neck, anterior and posterior	Sinus	Stomach	C1, 2, 3	Brow	Clavicular
Upper trapezius	Eye and ear	Kidney	C3	Crown	Ear
Supraspinatus	Brain	Conception	C4	Crown	Ear
Levator scapula	Parathyroid	Stomach	C5	Throat	Clavicular
Pectoralis major (clavicular)	Stomach	Stomach	C6	Throat	Shoulder
Pectoralis major (sternal)	Liver	Liver	C6	Throat	Clavicular
Biceps	Stomach	Stomach	C6	Throat	Elbow
Serratus anterior	Lung	Lung	C6	Throat	Shoulder
Subscapularis	Heart	Heart	C6	Throat	Shoulder
Infraspinatus	Thymus	Triple heater	C6	Throat	Shoulder
Brachialis	Stomach	Stomach	C6	Throat	Elbow
Brachioradialis	Stomach	Stomach	C6	Throat	Hand
Wrist extensors	Stomach	Stomach	C6	Throat	Hand
Triceps	Pancreas	Spleen	C7	Throat	Elbow
Middle and lower trapezius	Spleen	Spleen	C7	Throat	Shoulder
Supinator	Stomach	Stomach	C7	Throat	Hand
Latissimus dorsi	Pancreas	Spleen	C7	Throat	Intercostal
Wrist flexors	Stomach	Stomach	C7	Throat	Hand
Deltoid	Lung	Lung	T1	Throat	Shoulder
Teres major	Spine	Governor	T1	Throat	Elbow
Teres minor	Thyroid	Triple heater	T1	Throat	Elbow
Rhomboids	Liver	Liver	T2	Throat	Hand
Sacrospinalis	Bladder	Bladder	T2–L3	Heart	Intercostal
Abdominals	Small intestine	Small intestine	T4–T12	Solar plexus	Navel
Quadriceps	Small intestine	Small intestine	L1–2	Solar plexus	Groin
Iliopsoas	Kidney	Kidney	L2	Sacral	Groin
Sartorius	Adrenals	Triple heater	L3	Sacral	Knee
Gracilis	Adrenals	Triple heater	L3	Sacral	Foot
Tibialis anterior	Bladder	Bladder	L4	Sacral	Foot
Adductors	Circulation	Pericardium	L4–5	Sacral	Knee
Tensor fascia latae	Large intestine	Large intestine	L5	Sacral	Knee
Gluteus medius	Sexual	Pericardium	L5	Sacral	Groin
Gluteus maximus	Sexual	Pericardium	S1	Sacral	Knee
Hamstrings	Large intestine	Large intestine	S1	Sacral	Knee
Tibialis posterior	Adrenals	Bladder	S1	Sacral	Foot
Peroneus longus	Bladder	Bladder	S1	Sacral	Foot
Gastrocnemius and soleus	Adrenals	Triple heater	S2	Sacral	Foot
Popliteus	Gall bladder	Gall bladder	S3	Sacral	Knee

must be known. Secondly, it will be noticed that, with a few exceptions, the majority of the muscles have either the throat or sacral major chakra as a balancing point. The upper body muscles are associated with the throat chakra and the lower body muscles with the sacral chakra. These two points are accessed through their anterior aspects, namely the sternal notch (throat chakra) and a point three fingers' width below the umbilicus (sacral chakra or hara). The minor chakras are very easy to find, and their positions are listed in Table 3.3. There are also relevant Figures in the last two chapters showing the treatment of the muscles' involvement with the underlying pathology.

Relationships of the peripheral joints

The following section of this chapter will deal with the many reflected points and pathways of the peripheral joints. It is hoped that knowledge of these now will make it easier for the reader to understand the sections on treatment later on. Each peripheral joint has several reflected points that can be used for both analysis and treatment. These are situated on the ear, foot, hand, zone and parallel area. Whenever there is imbalance in the peripheral joint (pain, inflammation etc.), the reflected point will be tender. The more acute the condition, the more tender will be the reflected point. The more chronic the condition of the joint, the more diffuse will be the discomfort, and it will be impossible to 'rub the pain away' as it is sometimes possible to do in acute conditions. The ear reflexes are mostly used in analysis and diagnosis, as it is sometimes not practical to massage the ear – although, if it can be done, it can have great rewards. Most therapists, though, seem to treat the ear reflexes with needles (auriculotherapy). When it comes to treatment of the peripheral joints using the reflected points, the whole essence of the treatment is balancing of energy. This theme has been mentioned time and time again, but it is the cornerstone on which acupressure is built.

The reflexes are there to guide and aid us, but can be powerful tools when it comes to energy balancing. To do this, the therapist must first place the middle finger pad of one hand on the most acute (or painful) aspect of the joint to be treated and let it rest *in situ* for a few seconds, remembering not to use too much pressure. The middle finger of the other hand is then placed on one of the reflected points (ear, foot, hand, parallel or zone), and the therapist waits until there is a similar sensation under both fingers. This may take up to a couple of minutes to achieve. As has been stated many times before, there must be no hurry or attempt to rush the procedure on; the reflexes will be balanced in their own time and not before. Also, it is important that the therapist remains aloof to what is happening to the energy quality of the patient – after all, it is the patient's energy system that is being used, not the practitioner's. Concentration is necessary at all times, plus the ability to know when an energy balance has occurred, but the therapist must *not* allow his or her own energies to get involved!! When balancing has been achieved, the finger is placed upon the other reflexes in turn, whilst the 'local' finger remains still. After all the reflexes have been balanced, the joint should feel less painful and more in harmony with its surrounding tissues. The main thrust of the treatment may then take place, even though what has been done so far is usually more than half the battle towards achieving homoeostasis.

Each of the peripheral joints will be dealt with briefly below. The treatment procedures for specific conditions appertaining to the joints will be given in Chapter 7.

Reflexes of the temporo-mandibular joint (TMJ)

1. There is a very important stretch reflex on the middle of the forehead between the eyes that can be used before balancing is commenced. This has the advantage of relaxing the joint before the finger is placed on it.
2. There are two specific distal pain relief points associated with this joint, TH 5 and Con 17. These are used in addition to the reflex points. When the TMJ is in an acutely painful state, point TH 5 is an excellent distal point to use in order to balance the energy. There are often emotional aspects connected with tense TMJs, and the distal point of Con 17 is therefore an excellent point to use. (This point represents the anterior aspect of the heart chakra.)
3. The foot reflex is situated at the medial aspect of the great toe. This can be a very painful reflex in TMJ syndromes, and as such is used extensively in reflexology. The hand reflex is situated on the medial aspect of the thumb, and the ear reflex is on the lower posterior aspect, just above the lobe (Figure 5.7).

Reflexes of the shoulder joint

1. As mentioned in a previous chapter, the parallel area of the shoulder is the hip area. It is sometimes difficult to find an acute-

Figure 5.7   Reflexes of the temporo-mandibular joint.

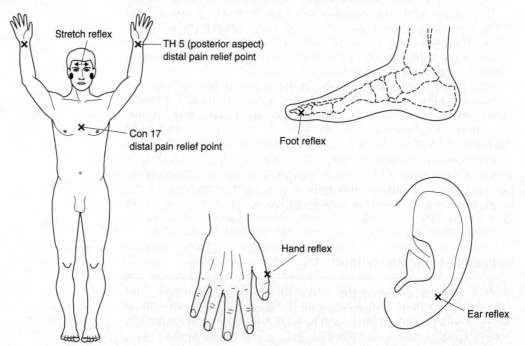

Stretch reflex

TH 5 (posterior aspect)
distal pain relief point

Con 17
distal pain relief point

Foot reflex

Hand reflex

Ear reflex

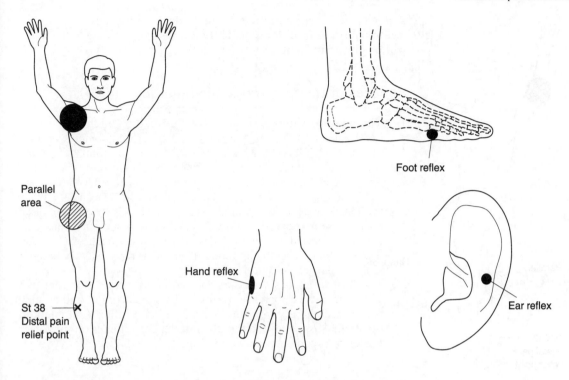

Parallel
area

St 38
Distal pain
relief point

Foot reflex

Hand reflex

Ear reflex

Figure 5.8 Reflexes of the shoulder joint.

ly tender point around the hip when there is a shoulder condition, simply because it is such a large area, but with perseverance one should be found.

2. There is a very useful distal point to use in shoulder conditions, namely St 38. This point is situated exactly halfway down the lateral aspect of the leg between the head of fibula and the lateral malleolus. In painful shoulder conditions, acute or chronic, this point is always tender, and represents an excellent distal balancing point, often giving seemingly miraculous relief of shoulder pain.

3. The foot reflex is situated at the distal end of the lateral aspect of the fifth metatarsal. The hand reflex is on the lateral aspect of the fifth metacarpal and the ear reflex is situated towards the posterior aspect of the ear.

It is interesting to note that there will always be a tender reflex of a painful peripheral joint, even though the joint in question may be mechanically or pathologically sound. In other words, even if the joint is painful due to a referred pain or aetiology elsewhere, the reflex will always be tender.

Reflexes of the elbow joint

1. The parallel reflex of the elbow joint is the knee. Generally speaking, if there is discomfort on the medial aspect of the elbow (e.g. golfer's elbow), there will be a tender reflex point on the lateral aspect of the knee; likewise, painful conditions of the lateral

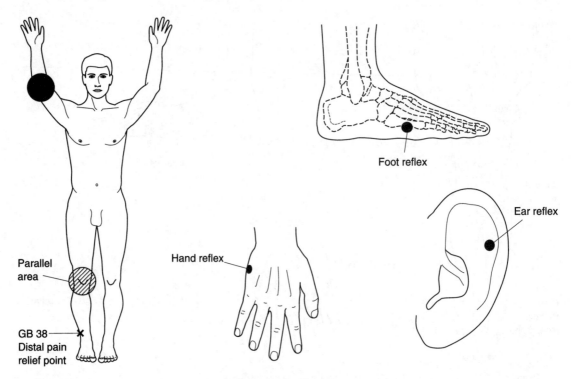

Figure 5.9   Reflexes of the elbow joint.

aspect of the elbow (e.g. tennis elbow) will give a painful reflex on the medial aspect of the knee.

2. The very useful distal point for pain relief is at GB 38. This point is exactly halfway between the reflex point of the shoulder (St 38) and the lateral malleolus.

3. The foot reflex is approximately halfway along the medial aspect of the fifth metatarsal. The hand reflex is halfway along the medial aspect of the fifth metacarpal and the ear reflex is just above the shoulder reflex at the posterior aspect of the ear (Figure 5.9).

Reflexes of the wrist joint

1. The parallel area to the wrist joint is the ankle. The palmar aspect of the wrist is associated with the posterior aspect of the ankle, and the dorsal aspect of the wrist is associated with the anterior aspect of the ankle.

2. The foot reflex is situated on the lateral aspect of the foot between the upper end of the calcaneus and the lower end of the talus. The hand reflex is situated on the dorsal aspect of the hand in the web between the fourth and fifth metacarpals, and the ear reflex lies just above the elbow reflex in the scaphoid fossa part of the ear (Figure 5.10).

Reflexes of the hip joint

1. The parallel area of the hip joint is the shoulder. There is nearly always a gnawing frontal shoulder ache with hip arthritis. A

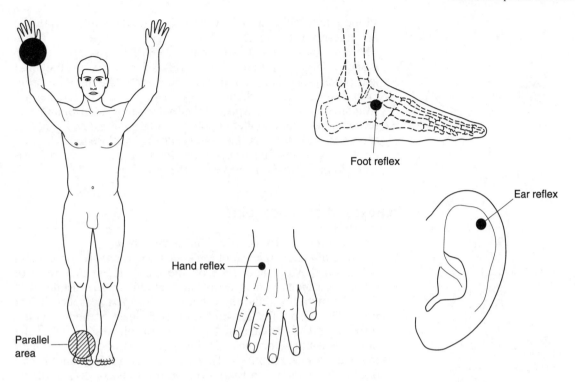

Foot reflex

Ear reflex

Hand reflex

Figure 5.10 Reflexes of the wrist joint.

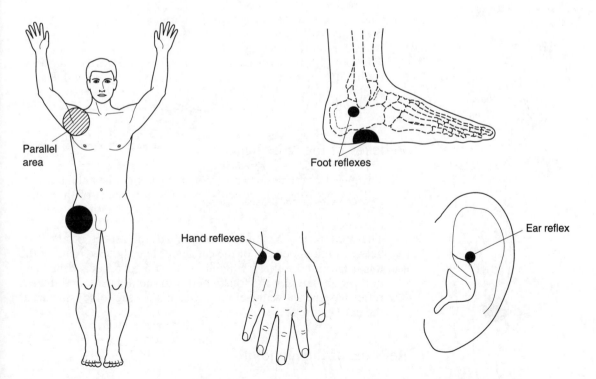

Parallel
area

Foot reflexes

Ear reflex

Hand reflexes

Parallel
area

Figure 5.11 Reflexes of the hip joint.

slipped femoral epiphysis will give a tender reflex over the acromio-clavicular joint.

2. There are two foot and two hand reflexes. This is because the hip is such a large joint that there are reflexes to represent the inner and outer aspects of the hip – in other words, the hip joint proper and the greater trochanter of the femur. The foot reflexes are situated on the lateral aspect of the foot, one just inferior and posterior to the lateral malleolus and the other one below the lateral aspect of the calcaneus. The hand reflexes are close to each other on the postero-medial aspect of the wrist crease. The ear reflex is situated at the antihelix aspect of the ear (Figure 5.11).

Reflexes of the knee joint

1. The parallel area to the knee joint is the elbow.
2. Because of the complexity of the knee joint, there are three reflex points on the foot and three on the hand. There are two foot reflexes on the lateral aspect of the foot, one on the distal end of the fifth metatarsal and the other on the superior aspect of that bone. The third reflex lies on the medial aspect of the foot at the forward end of the calacaneus. The hand reflexes are all on the dorsal aspect, two on the little finger and one on the thumb near to the anatomical snuffbox. There are also two reflexes in the ear, one in the scaphoid fossa and one in the superior crus antihelix (Figure 5.12).

Figure 5.12   Reflexes of the knee joint.

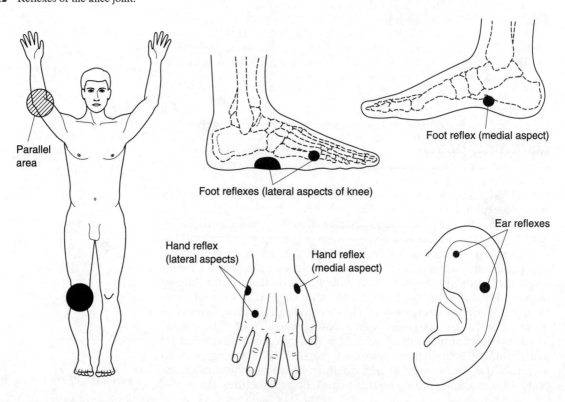

Parallel area

Foot reflexes (lateral aspects of knee)

Foot reflex (medial aspect)

Hand reflex (lateral aspects)

Hand reflex (medial aspect)

Ear reflexes

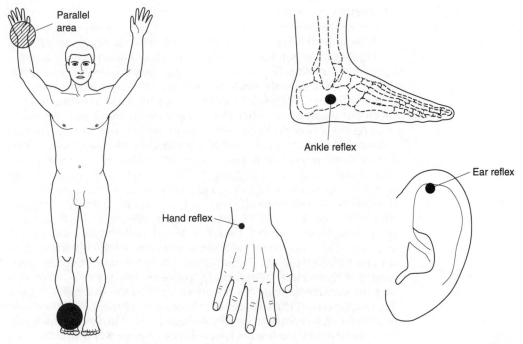

Figure 5.13   Reflexes of the ankle joint.

The ankle joint

1. The parallel reflex area of the ankle is the wrist.
2. The foot reflex of the ankle joint is situated on the lateral aspect of the foot in the middle of the calcaneus. The hand reflex is situated on the posterior wrist crease towards the medial end and the ear reflex is situated high in the superior crus antihelix (Figure 5.13).

Listening posts

This chapter concludes with the topic of listening posts as used in musculo-skeletal acupressure. The term 'listening posts' comes from cranio-sacral therapy, and is used to ascertain the quality and quantity of cerebrospinal fluid in a given system of the body – spine, soft tissue, joints etc. The usual areas of the body that are used as listening posts in cranio-sacral therapy are the occiput and the ankle. Cranio-sacral therapists are taught to place both hands on the occiput (known as the vault hold) or the ankles and 'tune in' to the flow of cerebrospinal fluid or energy flow. This technique can take months to master, and is an extremely subtle but powerful tool. The author learnt this technique several years ago and has since adapted it by using isolated acupuncture points on the skull as listening posts to ascertain the energy quality and quantity in various systems of the body – for example, the endocrine glands, bony structures etc.

Method

With the patient lying supine and the head comfortable on a soft pillow, the therapist sits behind the patient's head and slowly introduces the pads of the middle fingers to the various points as described below. After a few seconds, the emphasis of touch changes into an easier harmonious feeling. Nothing else will happen until the shift of emphasis of touch has taken place. After this change, the therapist has to concentrate on the aspect of the patient's energy system that is under analysis – this can either be a whole system, e.g. blood circulation, or can be narrowed down as much as is needed. This method of energy analysis has often been called 'finger dowsing' by practitioners. It is not something that will 'click' with therapists straight away; it takes time to master but, once mastered, can provide a very useful tool in analysis. The therapist simply 'asks questions' of the patient's energy system. This is done purely by thought, and not out loud. It is always best to gauge the overall energy picture of a system and then start to ask specific questions concerning individual joints, ligaments etc., rather than starting the questioning with specifics. What usually happens during this procedure is that the sensation under the fingers changes as the questions change. There appears to be a 'stillness' of movement in chronic conditions, and much heat and 'activity' in acute conditions. The reader is probably asking if these points are used only in analysis – the answer is that they can also be used in treatment of an energy imbalance in the system that is being dowsed. This is achieved by keeping the fingers *in situ*, concentrating totally on the system or body part that is in a state of imbalance, and gently twisting and turning to the movement of the energy flow whilst keeping the fingers on the points. It is helpful but not essential if the therapist has studied cranio-sacral philosophy, because this technique will then be second nature. The points below have proved to be useful in soft tissue and musculo-skeletal energy analysis, but represent just a fraction of what is possible with this philosophy (Figure 5.14).

Points used

St 2 – general energy

This point is situated in the depression in the infra-orbital foramen. The point is well known in many of the martial arts such as karate as a point that is stared at by an opponent to render the person weak. It is also used by exponents of 'touch for health' to create much the same effect. It is therefore an excellent point to use as a listening post to gauge the general energy system of the body. Once the shift of energy emphasis has been made and the therapist is working in an alpha–theta mode (see Chapter 4), questions can be asked about individual organs or joints. The energy quality will change under the fingers as the question is changed. As stated before, a dullness and stillness of energy flow under the fingers indicates that the body part is in a chronic imbalance, or Yin, and an increase of energy flow with obvious warmth indicates that there is an acute, or Yang, situation. The therapist can then proceed with some treatment and check the point afterwards to see if there is any change in sensation under the fingers. This goes for all the points.

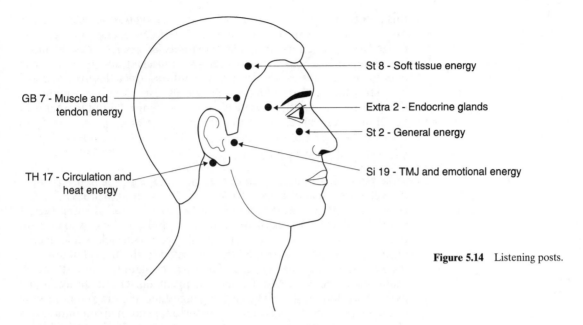

St 8 - Soft tissue energy

GB 7 - Muscle and
tendon energy

Extra 2 - Endocrine glands

St 2 - General energy

TH 17 - Circulation and
heat energy

Si 19 - TMJ and emotional energy

Figure 5.14 Listening posts.

St 8 – soft tissue energy

This point is situated 0.5 cun within the anterior hairline at the corner of the forehead. This point is a specific analysis point for soft tissue energy. The stomach energy is generally associated with soft tissue, and this point appears to be the best. Questions can be asked about the state of soft tissue, joints and skin, as well as the energy quality of the Earth element organs – the stomach and spleen. It is also an excellent point to ascertain the chronicity of rheumatoid and osteoarthritic joints.

Extra 2 – endocrine glands

This point is situated in the depression 1 cun posterior to the midpoint between the lateral end of the eyebrow and the outer canthus. This point is much used in cranio-sacral therapy as the point on the sphe-no-basilar synchondrosis to feel the 'movement' taking place in the sphenoid bone. In the middle of the two sphenoid bones lies the sella tursica, which houses the pituitary gland. As Extra 2 is the only point where any changes in sphenoid movement can be felt, it follows that it is of enormous value in gauging the energic quality of the pituitary gland. Once this has been felt, the therapist can then question the body about the energy state of the other endocrine glands. Hypo- or hyper-energic states of the endocrine glands will obviously affect the hormonal secretions of the glands and can have powerful influences on the general wellbeing of the patient, including the musculo-skeletal system. This point is also associated with the brow or third eye chakra, so is very influential in the treatment of pituitary dysfunction.

GB 7 – muscle and tendon energy

This is situated at the crossing point of the horizontal line of the auricle and the line that projects from the anterior auricle. In most people this point is quite tender. It is used as a listening post to ascertain the quantity and quality of muscular and tendinous energy. This can range from the general muscular capability of a person down to asking about specific muscles (or parts of muscles) and tendons. The energy influence is via the Wood element that rules the liver and gall bladder, which in turn affect muscle energy. There are other points on the liver or gall bladder meridians that can be used, but this seems to be the most effective.

TH 17 – circulation and heat energy

This point is situated posterior to the ear lobe, in a depression between the angle of the mandible and the mastoid process. This is a very influential point. It is said to be the ear chakra, which in turn is related to the heart chakra; it is therefore vital in emotions to do with the heart. Its main influence in the treatment of musculo-skeletal conditions is that it is said to be directly linked to the hypothalamus via the internal meridian system. The hypothalamus, amongst many other functions, deals with the heating mechanism of the body. When used as a listening post, TH 17 can gauge the wellbeing or otherwise of the blood circulation (arterial and venous) and the lymphatics. It is also, by questioning, able to give guidelines as to the cause of hot or cold conditions such as cold hands or feet.

Si 19 – TMJ and emotional energy

This point is situated in the depression shown between the tragus and mandibular joint when the mouth is slightly opened. As with all the other listening post points, this point is extremely useful and influential. It can be used locally to gauge the state of the temporo-mandibular joint. Its main claim to fame, though, is when used in acupressure as a calming point for emotional stress. It can therefore be used to great effect as a listening post for emotional imbalance. Care needs to be taken by the therapist when using this point as a listening post. It is such an influential point in the treatment of stress-related conditions that it is very easy to get carried away with concentrating on using it as a treatment point (which is all well and good when it is needed) to the detriment of using it as a listening post. The reader does not need to be told that many soft tissue and musculo-skeletal conditions have either emotional aetiology or emotional overtones. The purpose of this point when used in this way is to ascertain the cause of the underlying condition in checking whether or not it is emotional. This aspect of therapy and treatment is discussed fully in the book *Healing with the Chakra Energy System* (Cross, in preparation).

6

Principles of treatment

If the average Martian who has just landed on Earth were to ask an acupuncturist to define the noble art of acupuncture in two words, it would be an almost impossible task for the majority of acupuncturists. It seems very difficult to explain to any novice, including the average patient, exactly what acupuncture and acupressure is and how it works. It is all well and good to pontificate on the traditional or the many modern scientific theories, but sooner or later the enquirer will be baffled. The best definition that can be given is simply *energy balancing*. That two-word phrase sums it up in a nutshell.

Based upon the pain gate theory, science now has a working hypothesis to explain the effectiveness of acupuncture in pain relief. This has made the practice of acupuncture acceptable as an 'orthodox' therapy in the treatment of pain, and it is widely used for this purpose by both doctors and therapists alike. In a similar way the concepts of 'energy medicine' are also gaining increasing acceptance as the scientific evidence supporting this approach becomes ever stronger. It is to be hoped that energy medicine will become integrated into the mainstream of medical orthodoxy within the next decade, thus vindicating the holistic approach to patient care that is the very basis of this book and its philosophy. No apologies need be made for constantly referring to energy and to energy healing. These concepts lie at the heart of holistic medicine, and are gaining increasing verification from science.

Magnetism of the fingers

It has been mentioned several times, in different types of acupressure, that the practitioner places the *middle* finger of one hand on a point and the *middle* finger of the other hand on another point and then proceeds to balance the energy flow between them. Is it important to use these two fingers, and what is the significance in choosing them?

Figure 6.1   Magnetism of the hand.

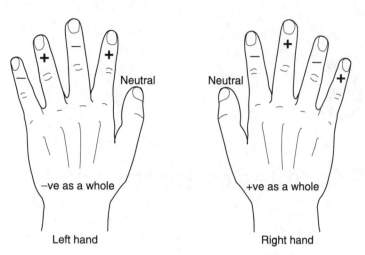

'Touch' therapists have argued for the past few decades about which fingers are used in their particular discipline, and have given several reasons for the relative values of using the correct fingers. The author can only write from his own experience of using many different disciplines of 'touch' therapy and draw relative conclusions from this.

It is said that each finger possesses either a negative or positive magnetic charge (Figure 6.1). The charge of the thumbs is said to be neutral and they therefore have little influence in subtle energy balancing, although great significance in practical acupressure. The flow of electricity and magnetism is said to go from the negative pole towards the positive pole. This certainly appears to be the case in the human body. It appears that one side of the body has a negative magnetic charge and the other has a positive one. One whole hand is negatively charged and the other is positive. So it follows that, in order to create a balance of energy between two points, it is better for the therapist to hold with two fingers that have an opposite charge in order that energy may flow more easily. If it is impossible to use the same two fingers, the balancing and hence the treatment will still proceed, but at a slower rate. The magnetism of the fingers does not matter when the energy balancing is done on the etheric level.

Energy flow and balancing

It follows from the previous section that one of the main principles of acupressure is the balancing of energy between two points. It is stated again, as it was earlier in the book, that the energy that is used is the patient's *own* vital force. There is absolutely no question of therapists utilizing their own vital force, nor are they 'channels' of healing as in reiki and spiritual healing. Balancing of Ch'i energy creates energy flow through a lesion, thus improving blood flow and lymphatic drainage to the area. Balancing of energy flow can take place along zones, meridians, reflexes, chakra points or great points.

General principles of treatment

Acute conditions

1. The local traumatic area, or lesion, needs to be sedated by placing finger(s) on suitable points adjacent to the lesion and allowing the inflammation to subside.
2. Suitable acupuncture points proximal and distal to the lesion are balanced in order to create a flow of energy through the lesion so as to create homoeostasis in the area.
3. It is essential that the cause of the acute lesion is treated in cases where the injury or lesion is not brought about by a direct blow. For example, in persistent hamstring tearing in athletes the acute lesion can be treated successfully by following the two points above, but unless the reason for the persistent tearing is not addressed it will happen again (this will be discussed further in Chapter 7). There are no shortcuts to the above procedure, it sounds longwinded and involved but, in practice, takes very little time.

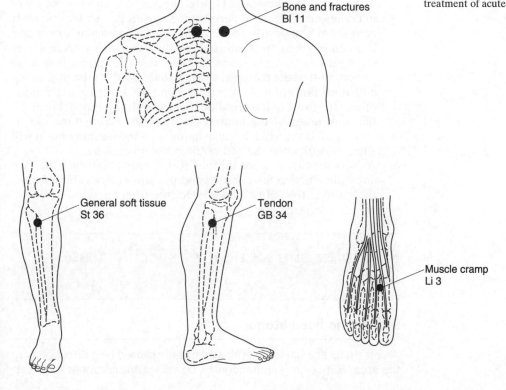

Figure 6.2 Important points used in the treatment of acute and chronic injuries.

Bone and fractures
Bl 11

General soft tissue
St 36

Tendon
GB 34

Muscle cramp
Li 3

Chronic conditions

1. It is essential in all cases of chronic conditions that a suitable distal acupuncture point is stimulated. This could be on the same meridian, zone or a chakra point. It must be a powerful point, and one of the great points. It is important in all cases of chronic injuries and musculo-skeletal conditions to 'create' Ch'i so as to have a reservoir of energy in order to support the healing process. It is never enough in chronic conditions, where there is energy depletion anyhow, to simply place the fingers on acupuncture points in order to treat; it will not happen! Energy has to be created in what is essentially a non-energic area.
2. The local lesion needs to be stimulated in order to bring more energy to the area. If, however, there is a sub-acute condition (mix of Yin and Yang) and the area is very painful, local points around the lesion need to be sedated whilst alternating with gentle stimulation. It is adequate gently to stimulate the point for a few seconds and to sedate for about 30 seconds.
3. Using suitable points both distal and proximal to the lesion, these are held for anything up to 2 minutes in order to create a flow of energy through the lesion.
4. The chronic lesion needs now to be supported energically by utilizing all the associated reflexes, zones and great points. This is done by placing one finger on the lesion whilst placing the same finger of the other hand on the associated points in turn, obtaining an energy balance in each case.
5. Finally, it is sometimes appropriate to place both hands around the injured part – if this is anatomically possible – and allow 'unwinding' to take place. Unwinding is a well-known procedure in cranio-sacral therapy, zero balancing and Bowen technique. It consists of allowing the twists and turns of muscular spasm and ligamentous tension to unwind, and the therapist merely places the hands around the lesion and lets this take place. It is most important that the therapist 'goes with the flow' of the unwinding and does not attempt to go the opposite way. This technique often affords incredible results. It must be firmly stated, however, that unwinding of the injured area will not be anything like as effective if done 'cold' at the beginning of the treatment as it will when performed at the end of the other procedures.
6. As with the case of acute injuries, it is essential that, once the pain and inflammation have settled and the area is more comfortable, the cause of the injury is addressed (see Chapter 7).

Principles of treatment of specific acute injuries

Soft tissue haematoma

A soft tissue haematoma (bruise) is usually caused by a direct blow to the area. If it occurs spontaneously, be very cautious about the treatment; it could be caused by a more serious problem such as a deep circulatory condition. It would be advisable for the patient to consult a GP if this were the case. The use of acupressure in acute injuries does not mean that the tried and tested orthodox physiotherapy treatments using ice, compression and elevation have to be avoided. On the contrary, it is essential that the area is cooled in order to prevent more bleeding into the tissues, supported by carefully applied bandaging to prevent the spreading of the haematoma and to afford comfort, and elevated as much as possible in order to prevent the formation of oedema. It is the author's experience that nothing is achievable with acupressure within the first 24 hours of the haematoma, as the risk of further bleeding into the tissues is too great if any kind of massage, however gentle, is performed. It is important, therefore, that the patient is instructed to use ice, compression and elevation (ICE) before any acupressure is attempted.

1. The area will be very painful, red and possibly swollen, so it may not be possible to perform any localized touch therapy or massage. If it *is* possible to do it, then simple finger-pad massage around the lesion is recommended in order to aid dispersal of fluid and to help with lymphatic congestion. If it is also possible to place fingers onto the bruise without too much pain, this should be done using very gentle pressure, slowly increasing the pressure as the comfort of the patient allows. *Never* push fingers into a haematoma quickly; you will not be helping the healing process at all – in fact, quite the opposite. Many a chronic condition has been caused by bad management of acute injuries, and what is done in first aid mode may determine the whole outcome of a sportsperson's career!! If it is impossible to place the fingers into the lesion site, gently place the whole hand over the injured area and massage exactly the same area on the other limb. This is a type of parallel acupressure, and is usually quite effective in initially relieving the acute pain and tension in the area. Whichever method is used, it will soon be found that the injured area is more comfortable and it is possible to proceed to the next stage of treatment.
2. The first stage was to disperse or sedate the excess Yang energy in the area. The next stage is to allow Ch'i energy to flow through the lesion and thus start to bring about homoeostasis in the area. Choose a point that is either a great point, command point or minor chakra point and is distal to the lesion (examples on the arm would be LI 4, TH 5, P8, and on the leg would be Bl 62, Sp 4 or Ki 1 – there are many more). It is not essential that the point chosen is on the same meridian as the lesion, but it will aid healing if it is. This point will have to be gently stimulated for a few moments. Then place the same finger of the other hand on a point proximal to the lesion – again, this point may need to be gently stimulated for a while. Then keep the fingers quite still. It will become apparent after about half a minute or so that a change of emphasis has taken place under the fingers and a balance of energy has occurred. The longer the acupressure balance is held, the more comfortable will be the injured area.
3. The next stage is to support the injured area energically by balancing the injured part to all its associated reflexes. The reflexes

on the hand, foot, skull or even ear could be used. It is also possible to use the parallel point on the opposite limb, or a point along the same zone. There are many different energy balances that can be done in order to heal the lesion. This will not, however, all be achieved in one treatment, and it would be advisable to see the patient for a follow-up session 2–3 days later. A specific point that can be used in the treatment of soft tissue lesions is St 36. It is well known in Chinese medicine that the stomach and spleen meridians are used to treat soft tissue conditions, and of all the points it is St 36 that seems to be the most powerful. This point is simply balanced with the site of the lesion, using St 36 on the same side of the body as the injured part.

Tendinitis

The treatment of acute tendinitis is very similar to the treatment of a soft tissue lesion, as is the treatment of a ligamentous strain; the exception is that the specific point used in all cases of tendinitis is GB 34. This point should be used as a balancing point with the lesion site during the treatment. In Chinese medicine the gall bladder meridian is associated with tendons, and experience has shown that this point is the most effective one to use. Treatment procedure for specific areas of tendinitis will be given in Chapter 7.

Muscle tears

Muscle tears are very common, and the sports physiotherapist will spend much of his or her time in their treatment. Usually this is done with ultrasound or another type of electrotherapy, coupled with massage of the area and stretching of the muscle so as not to encourage the formation of scar tissue following the inter- or intra-muscular haematoma that occurs when the muscle tears. As with the treatment of any soft tissue lesion, the principles of ice, compression and elevation should be adhered to, and it is not wise to commence any type of acupressure for at least 24 hours following the injury. The same procedure as for the treatment of a soft tissue lesion is carried out, with the following additions:

1. After balancing using a distal and proximal point in order to create a flow of Ch'i through the lesion and holding the points for a few seconds, it is very useful to massage between the two points using slow and deep strokes. It is helpful if the same sensation that the therapist felt under the fingers whilst holding the points is maintained as the massage is done. The massage should be very slow and performed with massage oil. The massage stroke is done with just one finger, starting at the distal point and proceeding through the lesion towards the proximal finger, whilst the other stays on the proximal point. As the massage stroke nears the muscle tear, the sensation felt under the massaging finger will change because the energy flow within the muscle lesion is different to the normal muscle tissue. It is now important that the massage is stopped until the same rhythm or one-ness is achieved as

before. The massage stroke is then carried on. Do *not* do any deep massage within 48 hours of a muscle tear, as there will be a danger of spreading the haematoma. This procedure may also be carried out in a chronic muscle tear, and is very effective in aiding the healing process.

2. The command point used in each and every acute or chronic tear is Li 3. In traditional Chinese medicine, the muscles are ruled by the Wood element – i.e. the liver and gall bladder. It has been shown that the gall bladder meridian energy is more effective in the treatment of tendon conditions, whereas the liver meridian energy is more effective with muscle imbalance. Therefore at some time during treatment it is essential that Li 3 is stimulated, followed by the point being balanced with the muscle tear site. Whilst discussing Li 3 as an effective point in muscle conditions, this point is *the* definitive point in the treatment of cramp – not just calf cramp, but cramp anywhere in the body, including 'stitch' pains that occur when the person cannot get rid of lactic acid quickly enough. Point Li 3 should be sedated in the treatment of cramp and should never be stimulated in any circumstances; the cramp will be made worse if it is.

Fractures

The reader is probably thinking, surely it isn't possible to use acupressure in the treatment of fractures? In actual fact, it is extremely effective in reducing pain and enhancing healing of the fracture site. This statement is, of course, purely subjective. There has not been any research, and the evidence is purely anecdotal using the author's experience. The procedure is very similar to the treatment of a muscle tear, with the exception that the therapist does not massage through the area.

1. Choose a powerful distal point to massage so as to create a reservoir of energy in the area.
2. Balance this point with a point proximal to the fracture site in order that energy flows through the fracture site, thus aiding blood and lymphatic circulation.
3. If it is feasible, place a finger (or hand) on the fracture site and hold for a couple of minutes. Remember that this touch is extremely gentle. Never in any circumstances move the limb; it must be kept still and supported at all times. As with other procedures, note that there will be a lot of heat produced.
4. Balance the fracture site with the opposite limb at the same point (parallel acupressure), the associated foot reflex point (reflex acupressure), or the ear or hand if this is easier to do.
5. Finally, stimulate point Bl 11. This point is situated on the inner bladder line 1.5 cun lateral to the lower border of the spinous process of the first thoracic vertebra. This is one of the associated effect points mentioned in Chapter 3, and is the one that is useful in the treatment of bony conditions. The reason why it is so helpful is that it is associated with the parathyroid glands, which are responsible for calcium metabolism. In any fracture site, acute or chronic, it will be found that Bl 11 will be tender, showing that it

needs treatment. The point should be stimulated for about 1–2 minutes, and this should be followed by balancing the point with the fracture site. As point Bl 11 is a bilateral point with the two points fairly close together, it should be possible to stimulate both points at the same time. When using the point to balance, only the point on the fracture site side of the spine should be used.

Principles of treatment of chronic and sub-acute joint conditions

The treatment of joint conditions by acupressure has been coined 'Chinese physiotherapy' by the author. The phrase sums up the procedure very well, although it can also be used to describe the treatment of muscular and other soft tissue lesions as previously described. This chapter will describe the procedure of joint conditions in general terms, followed by the treatment of specific joint conditions in the next two chapters.

The flow of Ch'i (vital force) appears to be greatest at the extremities of the limbs, i.e. the hands and feet. This is where most of the powerful command points are situated. The flow of energy throughout the arms and legs is therefore influenced more at these points than any other. It is essential that the command points are stimulated in all chronic and sub-acute conditions so as to create a reservoir of energy.

The most effective points for treatment of joint conditions

Figure 6.3 shows the main points used in the treatment of joint conditions.

1. Hand – P 8. Situated in the very middle of the palm. This point is also known as the hand chakra.
2. Foot –Ki 1. Situated on the sole of the foot in the mid-line, two-thirds of the way up from the heel. This point is also known as the foot chakra.
3. Elbow – P 3. Situated in the middle of the cubital fossa just to the lateral aspect of the biceps tendon. This point is also known as the elbow chakra.
4. Knee – Bl 40. Situated in the middle of the popliteal fossa. This point is also known as the knee chakra.
5. Shoulder – LI 15. Situated at the anterior and inferior border of the acromio-clavicular joint, inferior to the acromion, when arm is in adduction. This point is also known as the shoulder chakra.
6. Hip – GB 29 and St 31. There are two points associated with the hip; GB 29 governs the lateral aspect and St 31 governs the anterior aspect. GB 29 is situated midway between the anterior superior iliac spine and the highest point of the greater trochanter of

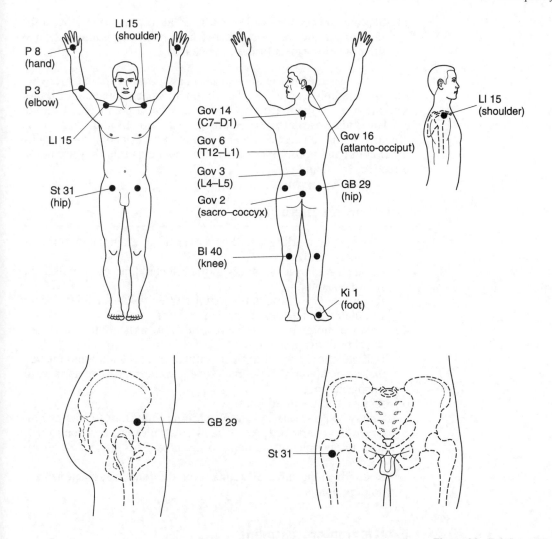

Figure 6.3 Points used in the treatment of joint conditions.

the femur; St 31 is situated directly below the anterior superior iliac spine, in a line level with the lower border of the symphisis pubis bone.

7. Upper cervical spine – Gov 16. Situated in a depression directly below the occipital protuberance, in the mid-line. This point is also the posterior aspect of the brow chakra.

8. Cervico-thoracic spine – Gov 14. Situated between the seventh cervical vertebra and the spinous process of the first thoracic vertebra in the midline. This point is also the posterior aspect of the throat chakra.

9. Thoraco-lumbar spine – Gov 6. Situated between the spinous processes of the twelfth thoracic and the first lumbar vertebra in the mid-line. This point is also the posterior aspect of the solar plexus chakra.

10. Lumbar spine – Gov 3. Situated between the spinous processes of L4 and L5 in the mid-line. This point is also the posterior aspect of the sacral chakra.

11. Sacrum and coccyx – Gov 2. Situated at the junction between the sacrum and the coccyx in the mid-line. This point is also known as the posterior aspect of the base chakra.

It can be seen from the above how many powerful points there are that the therapist can use in the treatment of painful and stiff joints. The majority of them are also known as chakra points (see Chapter 3). This indicates that these points are superior to and hence more effective than the usual command points. It is perfectly proper to use other command points, but experience has shown that they are not as effective. Try it and see!!

Order of treatment

1. Massage the meridians that pass over the joint, in the direction of the energy flow.
2. Create a reservoir of energy in the affected limb by stimulating a suitable distal point.
3. Balance energy through the joint between the distal point already stimulated and a suitable proximal point.
4. Balance energy between the painful area on the joint (lesion) and the chosen distal point.
5. Balance energy between the painful area on the joint and the various associated reflex points – zone, parallel, ear, foot, hand, skull or special point.
6. 'Unwind' the injured joint.
7. It may be necessary in suitable chronic conditions to massage the neuro-lymphatic reflexes (Chapman's reflexes) in order to help with the lymphatic drainage to the area. This stage isn't always needed.
8. Strengthen the muscles acting over the joint using acupressure holding points.

Explanation of treatment

1. It is essential that the therapist has as much of the patient's Ch'i as possible to utilize in the treatment. Therefore it is recommended that the treatment starts with meridian massage in order to boost Ch'i to the area. Where there is a sub-acute or chronic imbalance of the joint, the meridians are stroked in the direction of energy – the Yang meridians are stroked downwards and Yin meridians upwards. In the treatment of acutely painful joints, the massage is performed against the flow of energy. Meridian massage can even be performed through clothing if need be, although this is not recommended as later treatment will need work on the body.
2. In all cases of sub-acute and chronic joint conditions, the distal points have to be stimulated for at least a minute by using simple point stimulating massage. The more chronic the pain or condition, the more stimulation needs to be done. It is not important at this stage of the procedure where the other hand is placed, but usually it is comforting to place it on the painful joint. Experience

will tell how long the distal point needs to be stimulated; it varies from patient to patient and condition to condition, and is also dependent upon how much basic Ch'i the patient has. It is essential, though, that the therapist starts to get a 'feel' for what is happening underneath the finger that is stimulating the point. There should be an element of warmth that builds up after a few seconds and is often followed by a greater elasticity and softening of the tissues – even a 'putty' type of feeling. This sensation of altered awareness must be felt before proceeding to the next stage. The points used are P 8 in the palm for conditions of the arm, Ki 1 on the sole of the foot for conditions of the leg and Gov 2 between the sacrum and the coccyx for most spinal conditions (except that Gov 14, between C7 and T1, can be used if there is purely a cervical condition).

3. The next stage is to balance energy between the distal point (which has been stimulated and still has a finger on it) and an influential proximal point on the limb. The appropriate proximal point is located and held with the same finger of the opposite hand. Sometime the whole hand or a broad spread of several fingers is placed upon a large proximal area such as the sacrum or the shoulder. This is perfectly acceptable; at any stage, do what seems to be the most comfortable. The object of the exercise at this stage is to balance energy *through* the affected joint. This represents probably the hardest part of the whole procedure, and is especially difficult for beginners to this mode of healing. The over-riding principle is to let it happen and not to force or influence anything. The energy levels are bound to be sluggish if there is a chronic joint imbalance, so energy is not going to flow quickly and easily. Initially there may be a great divergence of sensation between the fingers; one may be pulsing warm whilst the other may be pulsing cold, or one may not have any sensation at all and the other may feel vibrant. Experience tells when the balance is complete, but the over-riding sensation is one of unanimity between the hands, there being a sensation that is the same under both fingers. A definite harmony is felt between one hand and the other. Often the patient will feel certain sensations such as warmth, trickling of water or even electric shocks. It is also important not to analyse too much of what is occurring in the patient's tissues. Make sure that energy balance has occurred before proceeding to the next stage.

4. The fourth stage is to balance energy between the powerful distal point and the painful area. This, of course, could be anywhere on the joint; it does not matter, so long as the finger(s) or hand is placed upon the painful area. This is, after all, where the symptoms are. As with most painful areas, care should be taken not to press too hard – light pressure is sufficient. After a few moments a similar sensation to that achieved in stage (3) will be felt. The 'hold' will probably be in the region of a couple of minutes, which is less than for stage (3), but here the therapist is capitalizing on the energy level that has been achieved so far and concentrating on where it is needed most – i.e. the chronic joint condition. It is useful to keep the fingers *in situ* for longer than is required to merely balance energy. The longer the fingers are held in place, the warmer and more pliable the tissues will become and the

more comfortable the whole area will feel. A change of emphasis should be felt during this stage, and it is at this point that the patient will start to feel the pain diminish.

5. It is now time for the next stage, which deals with supporting the energic quality of the injured part and also goes some way towards preventing further damage. The use of the associated reflex points is extremely important. The position of the various associated reflexes of the joints has been mentioned in the last chapter, so will not be covered again here. It is unimportant how many of the reflex or special points are used; the general rule is to use as many as the therapist is comfortable with in one treatment. Also, a particular kind of therapist will have different preferences – for example, a reflexologist would prefer to balance the painful joint with the foot reflex, whereas someone trained in head massage may prefer to use the skull reflexes. Practical comfort of the therapist also comes into the equation; it is not a good idea to have both arms at extreme stretch trying to stay relaxed, so use reflex points that are relatively close to the injured part! It may also be useful at this time to massage along the meridian with the flow of energy in order to bring more energy to the area.

6. This next stage of 'unwinding' may sound the most complicated, but in practice it is usually the easiest. In all trauma of joints and muscles there has been an acceptance by the body of a particular postural code that it is now exhibiting. It is well known that, when a joint is injured or arthritic changes start to occur, there are many postural changes that take place within the joint and the surrounding tissues as the remainder of the body adjusts to the new situation. In simple terms, the body attempts to protect itself from further damage – the surrounding ligaments and muscles become tighter and also assume the prime postural positioning according to the strength of the muscles acting around the joint. In order to 'heal' the joint (the word 'heal' simply means 'to make whole'), there must be a regaining of the original postural coding so as to allow comfort in the area and prevent further damage. In this final stage, therefore, there is simply an unwinding of this postural imbalance, which will finally bring about homoeostasis to the joint. This particular approach is well known to practitioners of cranio-sacral therapy, zero balancing and Bowen technique (to mention just three). The hands are placed on opposite sides of the joint and held for about 30 seconds. Warmth will then be felt and the joint will slowly unwind. This is a unique sensation to those practitioners who have not met it before, and it may take some time before it is mastered. Essentially what is happening is that with the aid of what has already been achieved in stages (1)–(5), the joint is attempting to return to normality in a subtle and yet very powerful way. Unwinding will not take place unless the joint has been prepared by earlier treatment. The golden rules in this procedure are exactly as have been stated several times before: let it happen and don't analyse it! The expression to 'go with the flow' is one that is often used, but it *must* be adhered to in this instance. The therapist is merely the instigator of a procedure that patients themselves carry out. Just sit back and let it happen!! All the therapist is doing is 'changing a gear' in the patient's energy field in order to facilitate self-healing! The

unwinding may take anything up to 5 minutes. It will also involve a change of hand positions so that all four 'corners' of the joint have been unwound. This old concept of naturopathic healing may seem a little strange for some readers, but have no doubt at all, this concept of energy medicine healing is the medicine of the future and one day will be accepted as standard procedure. It goes without saying that the more chronic the joint situation, the more treatments will be necessary in order to be successful.

7. In very chronic injuries where there is a lot of soft tissue sluggishness, fibrositis and fibrositic nodule formation, it is to be recommended that the Chapman's reflexes are massaged. The patient should be warned that this type of massage is not subtle, but can be quite heavy and sometimes painful. It seems to work very well though!

8. The final stage is to strengthen the overlying muscles with the help of the acupressure holding points. The therapist can also apply the triad of holding points, using the associated vertebral level and major and minor chakras. Do whatever is right for you and the patient. These procedures are explained in Chapter 5.

Procedures and points used for specific joints

The ankle joint

1. Stimulate the kidney, liver, spleen (Yin) vessels and the stomach, gall bladder and bladder (Yang) vessels.
2. Stimulate Ki 1 (sole of foot).
3. Balance the energy between Ki 1 and the knee (Bl 40).
4. Balance the energy between the painful area on the ankle or foot and Ki 1.
5. Balance the injured part with the associated reflexes.
6. Massage the Chapman's reflex.
7. Unwind the ankle or foot:
      dorsal aspect with palmar aspect
      medial aspect with lateral aspect.
8. Strengthen the gastrocnemius, tibialis anterior and peroneus longus muscles.

The wrist joint

1. Stimulate the heart, pericardium and lung (Yin) vessels plus three heater, small intestine and large intestine (Yang) vessels.
2. Stimulate P 8 (palm of hand).
3. Balance the energy between P 8 and the elbow (P 3).
4. Balance the energy between the painful area on the wrist and P 8.
5. Balance the injured joint with its associated reflex points.
6. Stimulate the Chapman's reflexes.
7. Unwind the wrist.
8. Strengthen the brachioradialis and wrist extensors and flexors.

The knee joint

1. Carry out meridian massage as per the ankle joint.
2. Stimulate Ki 1 (sole of foot).
3. Balance the energy between Ki 1 and the lower lumbar spine – L4–L5 (Gov 2).
4. Balance the energy between the painful area on the knee and Ki 1.
5. Balance the injured part to its associated reflex points.
6. Massage the Chapman's reflexes.
7. Unwind the knee:
   superior with inferior aspect
   medial with lateral aspect.
8. Strengthen the quadriceps, hamstrings, gastrocnemius and popliteus.

The elbow joint

1. Stimulate the meridians as with the wrist joint.
2. Stimulate P 8 (palm of hand).
3. Balance the energy between P 8 and the cervico-thoracic junction (Gov 14).
4. Balance the energy between the painful area on the elbow and P 8.
5. Balance the injured joint with the associated reflexes.
6. Massage the relevant Chapman's reflexes.
7. Unwind the elbow:
   anterior with posterior aspect
   medial with lateral aspect.
8. Strengthen the biceps, triceps and brachioradialis.

The hip joint

1. Stimulate the gall bladder, stomach and bladder meridians.
2. Stimulate either Ki 1 (sole of foot) or Bl 40 (behind the knee).
3. Balance the energy between Ki 1/Bl 40 and either L4–5 (Gov 3) or the sacro-coccyx junction (Gov 2).
4. Balance the energy between the painful hip point and Ki 1/Bl 40 (the painful point is often either GB 29 or St 31).
5. Balance the injured part with its associated reflex points.
6. Massage the associated Chapman's reflexes.
7. Unwind the hip:
   sacral region with the greater trochanter
   anterior hip area with the greater trochanter.
8. Strengthen the iliopsoas, gluteus medius, gluteus maximus and adductors.

The shoulder joint

1. Massage the large intestine, small intestine, gall bladder, three heater, lung, heart and pericardium meridians.
2. Stimulate either P 8 (palm of hand) or P 3 (cubital fossa).

3. Balance the energy between P 8/P 3 and the cervico-thoracic junction (Gov 14).
4. Balance the energy between the painful point on the shoulder and P 8/ P 3.
5. Balance the energy between the painful area and the associated reflex points.
6. Massage the associated Chapman's reflexes.
7. Unwind the shoulder:
    lateral aspect of shoulder with cervico-thoracic junction
    anterior shoulder with posterior shoulder.
8. Strengthen the deltoid, pectoralis major, triceps, latissimus dorsi, rhomboids, pectoralis minor and levator scapula.

The treatment procedures concerning spinal joints will be covered in Chapter 8.

Comfort of the therapist

This is something that is often overlooked by practitioners, but it is vitally important. Therapists often treat conditions that are caused by faulty posture. These conditions include low back pain, neck strain, headaches, repetitive strain syndrome and general tension. It is unusual for the therapist to admit that he or she is just as prone to acquiring these conditions as anyone else. With this type of work there could be several lengthy sessions of just holding two points, sometimes with outstretched arms, so it is imperative that every opportunity is taken to relax into the treatment. The following safeguards should prove to be handy:

1. Sit down whenever it is practical to do so.
2. Invest in a 'wheely' chair, thus making it easier to treat the patient and to continue from one set of holding points to the next without having to get up and move the chair. Also try and use a hydraulic couch so that the height may be adjusted.
3. When holding two points with either fingers or hands, don't be afraid of asking the patient if you can rest your forearms on them, thus relieving tension in the shoulders, neck and arms. The patient will not mind one bit.
4. Between treatments, get up and walk around or do some neck and low back stretching exercises.
5. Hygiene demands that the hands be washed between each patient seen. It is also a good idea to wash hands in running cold water. Although this type of 'healing' is nothing to do with spiritual healing or laying on of hands, nevertheless there could be some patients who exude negative 'vibes', and it is always best to safeguard oneself by washing the hands in running cold water.
6. Finally, learn to relax into the therapy. It is hard to do at first whilst learning the art, but this will become acquired as experience takes over.

7

Treatment of non-spinal musculo-skeletal conditions

The last two chapters of this book are devoted to the treatment of named musculo-skeletal conditions. Although acupressure will be the main treatment modality described, using techniques described in earlier chapters, it does not mean that all other physiotherapeutic procedures are null and void. Please do not assume that clinical acupressure is the be-all and end-all for every condition – it isn't. As was stated in the introduction, acupressure is a different approach, and can easily be incorporated (if applicable) into other treatment modalities. There is seldom an occasion when there is need to use *only* acupressure. It may well be found that the therapist has to perform a mix and match approach of combining different disciplines in order to give an holistic approach. Of course, these other approaches have to be learnt!! For instance, if the therapist is also an acupuncturist, reflexologist or cranio-sacral therapist, there is no reason why all these different approaches can't be utilized at the same time to give maximum effect. Also, please remember that the therapist can use subtle energy techniques until the cows come home, but if an underlying chronic joint fixation exists, often the only way to cure the patient is to move the joint. Of course, acupressure techniques will help provide the joint with Ch'i to make the adjustment easier, but acupressure alone will not adjust the joint (using either gentle or thrust techniques). Often it is the case that acupuncturists and acupressure therapists fall into the trap of assuming that their discipline will cure every musculo-skeletal condition alone – it will not. The best combination of skills is to be an acupuncturist and a manipulative therapist. This book has substituted acupressure for acupuncture in order to help purely hands-on therapists, but the theory is the same. Massage is equally important. Before acupressure is commenced, it is a good thing to massage generally around the area, thus increasing the blood flow to the area. The use of massage oil is recommended; the ideal base is one of soya oil, which can have a few drops of an appropriate aromatherapy oil added if necessary.

Order of treatment

Whatever the individual condition, there is a rough 'batting order' for treatment. That detailed below represents a rule of thumb, and may need to be changed for certain conditions.

1. Massage the overlying meridian (direction of flow in chronic conditions and against the flow in acute conditions).
2. Treat the points local to the lesion. Gentle stimulation is needed in chronic conditions, and sedation in acute conditions.
3. 'Create' energy at a suitable distal point. This can be a point on the distal end of the same meridian, a minor chakra point or a special point.
4. Balance Ch'i energy through the lesion.
5. Balance Ch'i energy between the lesion and the distal point.
6. Balance Ch'i energy between the lesion and the associated reflex (reflected) points.
7. Use special points and procedures pertinent to the lesion.
8. Unwind the lesion.

Temporo-mandibular joint (TMJ) syndrome

This is a composite of symptoms that affect this extremely important joint. The joint could have a slight subluxation due to trauma by being hit on the jaw or biting on something hard. It could have a chronic inflammation due to a misaligned jaw or constant teeth grinding. Symptoms of most of the above include joint clicking and pain. The pain is often referred towards to the shoulder on the same side, and there is often trigeminal nerve (and sometimes facial nerve) involvement.

The muscles that act on the TMJ and are responsible for its movement are the temporalis, masseter, internal pterygoid and external pterygoid. The buccinator is the principal muscle of the cheek and forms the lateral wall of the oral cavity, and as such it is an accessory muscle of mastication. All these muscles are associated with the stomach meridian (applied kinesiology), and the stomach meridian lies adjacent to the joint itself. Research has shown the TMJ to be associated with generalized body muscle distortion and also with stress-related conditions. Perhaps grinding the teeth is symptomatic of the stress that causes the condition in the first place. Cranio-sacral therapists and cranial osteopaths are well aware of the importance of the TMJ with regard to cranial dysfunction. Therefore, correct treatment of TMJ syndrome can have enormous ramifications on the wellbeing of both the physical and the emotional body.

Treatment

1. Massage the stomach meridian from the head to the toes (direction of energy flow). Care must be taken when stroking the

Figure 7.1 Points used in the treatment of temporo-mandibular joint syndrome.

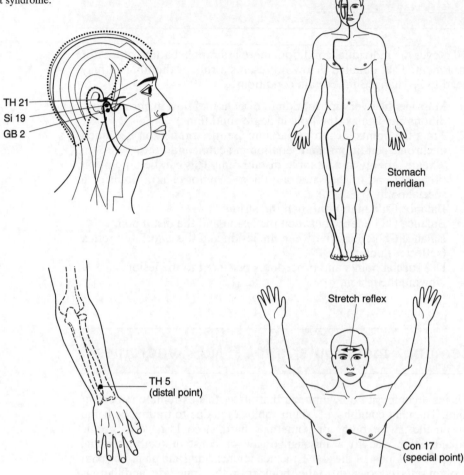

TH 21
Si 19
GB 2

Stomach meridian

TH 5
(distal point)

Stretch reflex

Con 17
(special point)

meridian on the face; this has to be done with finger pads, whereas the palm of the hand can perform the stroking on the rest of the meridian. This should be performed about three or four times bilaterally.

2. Do gentle stimulating massage to the points local to the TMJ – TH 21, Si 19, GB 2 and St 7 (Figure 7.1). Point Si 19 is perhaps the one that is most central to the joint, and is usually the one that is used in the later stages of the treatment.

3. The best distal point to create energy in the area is TH 5. This sounds slightly odd, as it is neither on the stomach meridian nor on the small intestine or gall bladder meridians, which also lie adjacent to the joint, although TH 21 lies to the superior end of the TMJ. It isn't even a chakra point. However, experience has shown that TH 5 is the best point. This should be massaged for about 2 minutes, until warmth has built up and it is obvious that energy is available for use.

4. Balance TH 5 with TH 21 to allow energy to flow through the joint. This may take up to 2 minutes and, if done correctly, a shift

of energy emphasis should take place. The joint should be feeling quite a bit more relaxed, even though it has not been touched.

5. The next stage is to use the stretch reflex, which is situated on the frontal bone on a horizontal plane about 3 cm up from the glabella. With the patient lying down, place the pads of the middle fingers on either side of the stretch reflex and gently part the fingers, thus stretching the skin apart in a horizontal plane. This should be done for about 2 minutes.

6. Now place the middle finger pad onto the painful aspect of the TMJ (usually point Si 19) and balance with TH 5. This will start to create much more relaxation in the joint and indeed in the whole area.

7. The associated reflexes may now be balanced with the joint. Try the foot or hand reflex, or even the ear reflex. These points are illustrated on Figure 5.7.

8. Now balance the lesion with point Con 17, which is situated in the middle of the sternum. This is particularly useful if the cause of the TMJ syndrome is anxiety and stress. Con 17 is the frontal aspect of the heart chakra, and is often used to release old stress situations that have manifested themselves as physical symptoms.

9. The unwinding of the joint is quite straightforward if there is just chronic inflammation and not subluxation. Simply place the finger pads on both TMJs for a few moments. Unwinding will soon commence with gentle sways of movement – remember to 'go with the flow'. If the joint was in a state of chronic inflammation, the treatment is now finished, although it may take another couple of sessions to complete the task. If the joint is subluxed, it is in a much more relaxed state to attempt a simple reduction. This, however, is a specialized skill that requires training, and is not to be carried out by untrained personnel. Any good osteopathic or chiropractic manual will explain it.

Sterno-clavicular joint pain

The sterno-clavicular joint forms a lynchpin between the shoulder girdle and the sternum, and is often injured through a fall on the outstretched hand or by a direct blow. As with the TMJ, there is a fibrous cartilage within the joint, so it can be prone to subluxation and even dislocation, thus giving great instability to the whole area. It is, sadly, a joint that is often ignored by therapists as being irrelevant, but when the energic considerations are taken into account, it is of profound importance. It lies very close to some very powerful points (Ki 27 and Con 22), and of course lies close to the important organs of the superior vena cava, oesophagus, thoracic duct and thyroid gland.

Treatment

1. The associated meridian is the stomach, as this is the only meridian that is situated close to the joint and has a superior and inferior influence anatomically. The meridian needs to be stroked in the direction of flow if the joint is in a chronic condition or against the flow if it is acute.

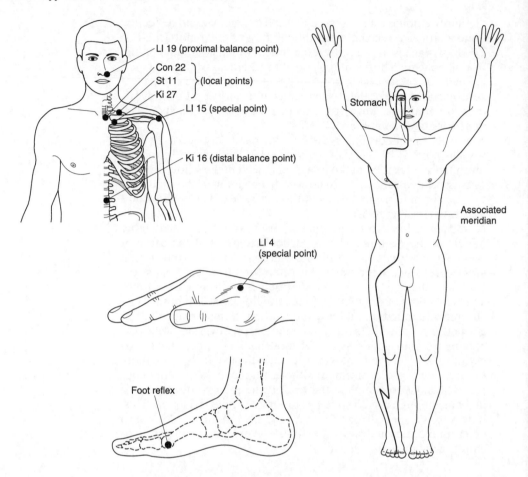

Figure 7.2 Points used in the treatment of sterno-clavicular pain.

2. Gently massage the local points of Con 22, Ki 27 and St 11 for a few seconds each (Figure 7.2).
3. A useful distal point to influence a build-up of energy is Ki 16. This point is situated adjacent to the umbilicus. One of the kidney points that lie in the intercostal spaces can be used; these are, of course, closer to the joint, but can be very tender to massage.
4. To balance Ch'i through the joint, it will be necessary to place the other finger on a non-kidney point (because the kidney meridian ends just below the clavicle). The ideal point would be Li 19, which is situated just below the nose; it lies in the same zone as Ki 16, hence its influence.
5. Balance the most painful part of the joint with Ki 16. This may take some time if the joint is in a chronic state.
6. The lesion may now be balanced with the suitable reflexes. The most effective one is on the foot, although the parallel point is useful.
7. The special points of influence are Li 15 (the shoulder chakra) and Li 4, which is useful in all painful conditions of the front of the chest and face.
8. Unwinding is carried out by placing one hand over the sterno-clavicular joint and the other hand over the cervico-thoracic junction. If there has been a subluxation of the joint the unwinding

will very often reduce it, but if it doesn't, then a very gentle anterior to posterior thrust is usually all that is needed to reduce the joint, thus saving the patient from ongoing pain and stiffness.

Acromio-clavicular subluxation and pain

The acromio-clavicular (A/C) joint is often subluxed due to a fall on the outstretched arm or the elbow. If not treated adequately whilst at first aid or in the first 24 hours following injury, it can be sometimes very difficult to reduce later on. A chronic AC joint subluxation can be very disabling, and has ruined many sporting careers. The joint should be taped almost immediately after injury (as well as giving ice, compression and elevation – ICE) to allow the internal fibrocartilaginous articular disc to remain stable.

Treatment

1. The associated meridian is the lung, and this should be stroked in the first instance. Only the meridian on the affected side need be stroked.
2. Do some gentle circular finger massage on the four local points, LI 15, LI 16, TH 14 and Si 10 (Figure 7.3). The first two are the most important, and it is usually the case that the lesion is exactly on LI

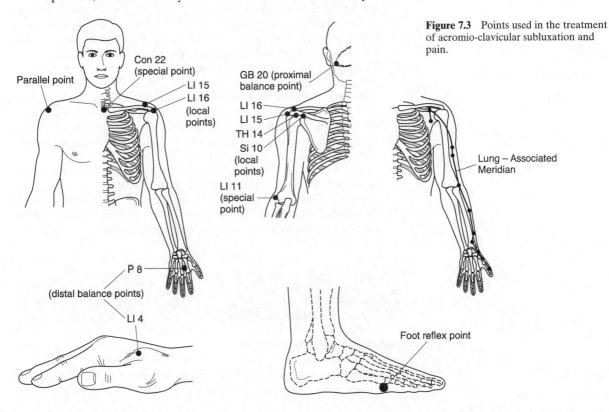

Figure 7.3   Points used in the treatment of acromio-clavicular subluxation and pain.

15. Remember to spend a little time on this initial massage in chronic cases. When the joint is acute, the points just need to be touched until heat and inflammation is felt being pulled away.

3. There are two possible distal points that can be used in order to create energy. Each has merits. Point P 8 (situated in the palm of the hand) is a minor chakra point and, as such, can be used as a distal point in most upper limb trauma. LI 4, on the other hand, lies on the same meridian as LI 15, but experience has shown that if LI 4 is stimulated too strongly it can affect the bowel!!! The best option is to use P 8 and keep LI 4 in reserve as a special point later in the treatment.

4. To balance Ch'i through the lesion, choose the proximal point of GB 20. This has a double effect. It is a powerful point in the relief of occipital pain (which often occurs with A/C subluxation), and it lies at the upper aspect of the trapezius muscle (the A/C joint is close to the middle fibres of the trapezius), thus allowing muscular relaxation.

5. Now balance the lesion (usually LI 15) with the distal point (P 8 or LI 4). Hold this for much longer than is required just to achieve a balance of energy under the fingers. This, without doubt, is the most comforting part of the treatment.

6. Place a finger on the lesion (usually LI 15) and balance with its associated reflexes. The most effective are the parallel point (on the other A/C joint) and the foot. For the foot reflex balance, the patient will probably have to bend the knee up so that the therapist can perform the balance and yet remain comfortable.

7. The special points that can be used are Con 22 (situated in the sternal notch), LI 11 (situated on the outside of the elbow joint at the end of the crease when the elbow is fully flexed) and LI 4 (between the thumb and first finger at the first interosseous muscle), if this point has not already been used as the distal balance point.

8. The joint is unwound by placing one hand over the joint and the other one over the cervico-thoracic junction (as per the sterno-clavicular joint). Some unwinding with the hands placed anterior and posterior to the joint may be needed. In the case of a mild subluxation, it should be easy now to ease the joint into alignment by giving a gentle downward thrust – once again, it is emphasized that this procedure may need specialist training. If the subluxation is a chronic one, it may require two or more sessions before reduction of the joint can be attempted. Whatever the state of the joint, it is always a good idea to reinforce the treatment by taping the joint down, thus allowing maximum healing time. A collar and cuff or broad arm sling is also recommended.

Shoulder conditions

Supraspinatus tendinitis

The supraspinatus tendon forms the upper part of the rotator cuff group of muscles that support and protect the non-congruous gleno-humeral joint. Inflammation of the tendon takes place either due to a series of repeated microtraumas to the area or by a prolonged stretch. The tendon can also be partially or totally ruptured – this would necessitate surgical intervention. Supraspinatus tendinitis is a very painful lesion and can affect the whole of the shoulder girdle, with muscles going into spasm due to the patient's self-protecting mechanism. Classical treatment of this lesion would include ultrasound, heat and transverse friction massage, which are beloved by many physiotherapists. This treatment regimen is very successful, but the procedure can be painful and may also give a slow response and recovery rate. Acupressure has enormous benefits in that it aids the patient's own healing mechanism, thus speeding up the healing process, and it is not painful.

Treatment

1. The associated meridian of the supraspinatus is the conception meridian. The study of applied kinesiology has linked this single small yet significant muscle to this meridian. Stroke the meridian in the direction of flow from the symphysis pubis to the chin (do not stroke near the mouth). This needs to repeated four or five times.
2. The local points are LI 16, which lies just over the insertion of the tendon at the humerus, and TH 14, which lies more on the musculo-tendinous intersection (Figure 7.4). These two points need to be gently massaged with the finger pads in a circular motion (like doing circular friction, only with much less pressure).

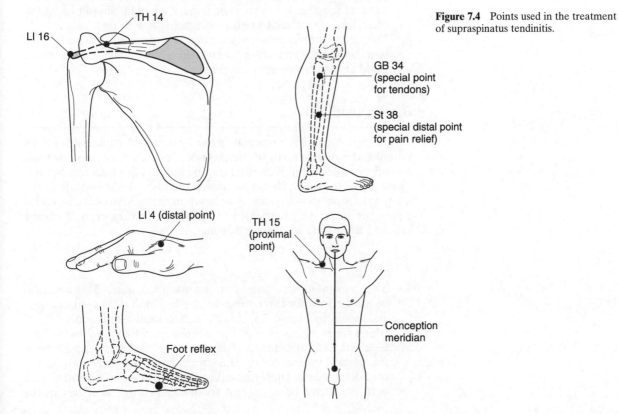

Figure 7.4   Points used in the treatment of supraspinatus tendinitis.

3. The distal point to create Ch'i is LI 4. Do not over-massage this point – as stated previously, it has wide-ranging effects. This point is forbidden to heavy massage in the early months of pregnancy, at menstruation, and if the patient has bowel looseness. Choose point P 8 in the palm of the hand if the patient has any of these conditions.

4. A good proximal point to choose is TH 15. This point is easy to find in that it lies exactly halfway between the point of the shoulder and the seventh cervical vertebra, just behind GB 21 (which would also make a useful proximal point). Stimulate this point and LI 4 together, and then balance the two so as to create a balance of Ch'i through the lesion. This may have to be done for up to 2 minutes before the energy flow can be felt.

5. Next, balance the most painful point on the supraspinatus (usually LI 16) with LI 4. In very acute conditions, much heat will be produced. Heat will also be produced in sub-acute and chronic conditions, but it will be slower to happen.

6. Now balance the lesion with its reflected points. The best ones are the exact same point on the other shoulder (parallel) and the foot reflex. The hand reflex also has its merits, and is easier to do practically (see Figure 5.8).

7. There is a special point, St 38, situated halfway between the head of the fibula and the lateral malleolus just forward of the fibula. This point is always painful in any shoulder condition, and can be used as an excellent distal pain relief point. The balancing of the lesion with St 38 is probably the most effective part of the treatment. The special point for tendons, GB 34, just forward of the head of the fibula, is also to be used. This point should be stimulated for a few seconds before balancing it with the lesion.

8. Unwinding of this lesion is not easy! It is probably best performed with one hand over the general area of the lesion and the other hand at the cervico-thoracic junction.

Biceps tendinitis

The biceps brachii is responsible for flexion and supination of the elbow and is also a flexor of the shoulder. The short head of biceps is sometimes affected in biceps tendinitis, but it is the long head that is more prone to strain. This is because it blends with the capsule of the glenoid labrum and also runs in a sheath in the groove of the humerus called the intertubercular sulcus; it is therefore very prone to being affected by repetitive strain syndrome.

Treatment

1. The associated meridian is the stomach meridian. This needs to be stroked two or three times in the direction of flow of energy.

2. As shown in Figure 7.5, there are five local points, only two of which are meridian points. The nearest meridian point to the long head is LI 15, whereas LI 16 is nearest to the biceps expansion at the gleno-humeral joint. The other three points are all 'extra' meridian points. These are called Taijian, Jianneiling and Chupi, with the latter being closest to the long head, as it lies in the

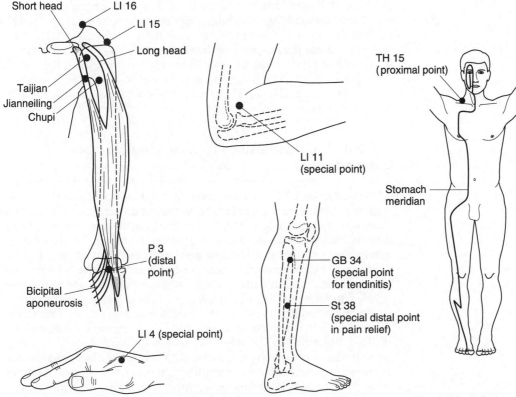

Figure 7.5 Points used in the treatment of biceps tendinitis.

humeral sulcus. These points need to be stimulated for a few seconds if the condition is chronic, and just held if it is acute.

3. The distal point for creating Ch'i energy is P 3, which is situated on the medial side of the insertion of the biceps tendon at the elbow. This point needs to be stimulated for anything up to 2 minutes in a chronic condition.

4. The proximal balancing point is TH 15, which is the same one as is used in the treatment of the supraspinatus. It is easily accessible, and balancing between it and P 3 creates a nice 'glow' around the shoulder that is very comforting to the patient.

5. Next, the painful lesion (wherever it is on the biceps origin) needs to be balanced with P 3. Keep this hold on for anything up to 3 minutes, as it will help to energize the area.

6. Now balance the lesion with its associated reflex points. These are the biceps origin on the opposite side (parallel) and the shoulder reflexes on the foot or the hand.

7. The special points used in biceps tendinitis are the most effective ones. First, it is important that point GB 34 is stimulated, as with all tendon injuries. Next, balance the lesion with the special point for pain relief around the shoulder, namely St 38, which is found halfway down the lateral aspect of the fibula. Also balance it with points LI 4 and LI 11. These two provide the most pain relief, and it is therefore more sensible to dwell on these two points for longer than required merely to create an energy balance.

8. Unwinding is done by placing the hands anterior and posterior to the shoulder complex, with one hand directly over the lesion. After unwinding, with the patient feeling comfortable, it is a good idea to use the acupressure holding points for the muscles associated with the stomach meridian in order to strengthen the muscle (Figure 5.6a). The points to be held are St 41 with Si 5, followed by St 43 and GB 41. This practice needs to be carried out after each session.

Chronic shoulder lesions (frozen shoulder and osteoarthritis)

The conditions of frozen shoulder and osteoarthritis of the gleno-humeral joint are a nightmare for doctors and therapists alike. There does not seem to be a standard treatment for these very painful conditions. Standard conservative treatment usually consists of heat, electrotherapy, gentle exercises and anti-inflammatory medication. Treatment by acupressure is definitive and accurate, with a very high success rate. The problem that the therapist has is treating the *cause* of the condition. If the patient says that the pain and stiffness started as a result of an injury around the shoulder or as a result of repetitive strain, then the conservative physiotherapy approach often works well. If, however, the patient informs the therapist that 'it just happened', the cause could be anything. As the reader is already aware, there are some important meridians that flow over the shoulder; namely the lung, large intestine, small intestine and triple heater. Chinese medicine tells us that these meridians all influence excretion in some form or another. If there is an energy block or stagnation arising in these meridians or associated organs, there is often a physical and emotional stagnation that can cause symptoms such as constipation, skin eruptions, catarrh and depression, among others. The shoulder is therefore merely the part of the body that houses the symptoms, and it is useless specifically to treat the shoulder without incorporating the holistic paradigm. This is explained more fully in *Healing with the Chakra Energy System* (Cross, in preparation). Clinical acupressure allows patients to heal themselves by having their Ch'i balanced. The symptoms will ease if the holistic principle is adhered to. Of course it is essential to ease the pain in the shoulder, because that is what the patient expects. With acupressure it is possible to both treat the pain and treat the whole!

Treatment

1. The meridians that flow over the shoulder are the large intestine, small intestine, lung and triple heater, with the pericardium and gall bladder meridians lying very close by. All these meridians need to be stroked with the flow of energy. Approximately two or three strokes on each meridian is sufficient.
2. The local points now need to be stimulated, and these are Lu 1, Lu 2, LI 15, LI 16, GB 21, Si 10, TH 14 and Si 9 (Figure 7.6). Not all the points need to be stimulated – only the ones that are pertinent or close to the pain. It is important however that, if there is any physical sluggishness, the points of the large intestine are

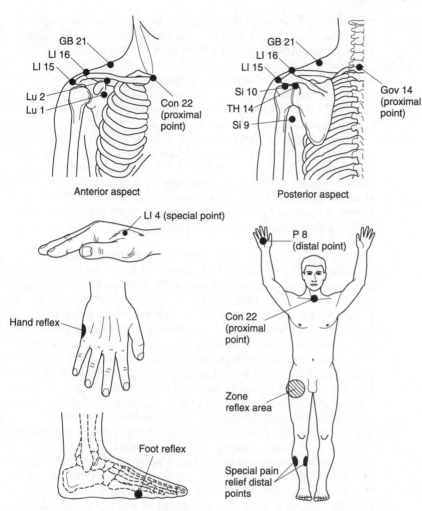

Figure 7.6   Points used in the treatment of chronic shoulder conditions.

stimulated. If there is any skin trouble or catarrh, then the two lung points should be stimulated. In all cases of depression and other emotional imbalance, GB 21 and TH 14 should be stimulated. Whilst the therapist is stimulating each point, it is important to note which ones are the most tender. This will give an indication of the type of chronic shoulder it is.

3. The most useful distal point to create Ch'i energy is P 8, situated in the middle of the palm. However, if there is an over-riding sluggishness in the patient's system, then LI 4 may be the better option. Whichever point is chosen, it needs to be stimulated for at least 2 minutes, breaking off from the stimulation just to hold the points occasionally to ascertain if sufficient energy for the therapist to work with has been produced. Experience is the only guide here.

4. To balance Ch'i through the lesion, the distal point of either P 8 or LI 4 needs to be balanced with points Con 22 or Gov 14. These are situated in the sternal notch and at the cervico-thoracic junction respectively. Con 22 is the anterior aspect of the throat

chakra, and Gov 14 is the posterior aspect. They are both very powerful acupressure points, and are particularly valuable in shoulder conditions. Because the major chakra points have influences with our aura and our emotional selves, they are often used to good effect in the treatment of physical conditions that have an emotional aetiology. Frozen shoulder may be such a condition, especially if there is no known mechanical cause. The throat chakra is associated with expression and the ability to express emotions easily or otherwise. If a patient cannot express emotions easily, a frozen shoulder can ensue after years of emotional frustration. A common expression is 'cannot shoulder responsibility'; another is 'has the world's worries on his shoulders'. Much study and research has been done in the field of relationships between body and emotions, and into body language. One of the author's main studies over the past few years has been in this field.

5. The therapist now has to balance the most painful aspect of the shoulder condition with the distal point. There may be more than one painful point, but always start with the most tender, as usually this is the one that is 'crying out' for treatment first. Once this painful point is rendered pain-free (it may take more than one session) others may become the tender points, but the over-riding principle at this stage is to work through the most painful point.

6. There are several reflex points for the shoulder that can be of help. The foot and hand reflexes are useful, especially the foot. Even the ear reflex has its merits. There is also the parallel point on the other shoulder – this point may need to be stimulated slightly before attempting an energy balance. The zone reflex area is at the hip. As the hip region can be such a naturally tender area, it is not always easy to ascertain a tender reflex, although there is always one there. Usually, if the lesion is on the anterior aspect of the shoulder, the tender reflex point will be on the front of the hip. If the tender point is on the lateral aspect of the shoulder, the tender hip point will be on the lateral side, and so on.

7. There are a few special points that can be useful. First, there is the great pain relief point of LI 4. This can be used here as well as using it as a distal point. There are also the special distal pain relief points that lie on the leg halfway between the knee and the ankle. Once again, as with the hip reflex, if the shoulder is painful on the lateral aspect, the painful reflex will be on the lateral aspect of the leg (normally St 38). If there is a medial pain or one that affects the whole of the shoulder girdle, the reflex will be tender on the medial aspect of the leg, normally at Sp 6. It is just a question of feeling for it – it will be there. As before, this aspect of the balancing will produce the most effective results, and the patient often exhibits a great deal of pain relief at this stage. This, obviously, will be accompanied by more movement in the shoulder girdle. Again, it is emphasized at this stage of the procedure, please allow things to happen and do not will anything to happen. During the first treatment of a very chronic shoulder, hardly anything will happen, because the situation is so chronic and long-standing and the energies are so deep that it takes time and effort to raise them.

8. The shoulder can be unwound in two ways. First, place one hand on the lateral aspect of the shoulder and the other at the cervico-thoracic junction. Secondly, place one hand on the front and the other hand on the back of the shoulder.
9. Two useful procedures to finish a treatment session are as follows:

    Massage the meridians just around the shoulder. This can be done with more pressure than at the beginning of the treatment. Connective tissue massage can be used, but please warn the patient that it will be 'stimulating'.

    Massage the Chapman's reflexes around the area. The ones around the clavicle, sternum and down the cervico-thoracic spine are particularly useful.

Elbow conditions

Tennis elbow

This condition is one of muscular and tendinous overstrain due to excessive strain of the wrist extensors, such as in prolonged use of the backhand in tennis. The onset is nearly always gradual. There are at least three types:

1. Myositis or fibrositis of the brachioradialis muscle at either the belly of the muscle or the muscular tendinous intersection.
2. Periostitis in the region of the lateral epicondyle, with actual tearing of one of the wrist extensors from its periosteal attachment.
3. Synovitis of the superior radio-ulnar joint.
    These three can be seen together or individually.

Treatment

1. The brachioradialis and extensor digitorum muscles are associated with the stomach meridian. This needs to be stroked in the direction of energy flow. The meridians that flow near to the lesion site need also to be stroked, i.e. the large intestine and lung. These just need to be stroked on the painful arm.
2. There are four main local points, three of which are on the large intestine meridian – LI 10, LI 11 and LI 12 (Figure 7.7). Lu 5 is the other local point. These points need to be stimulated in the case of a chronic lesion and sedated in the case of an acute lesion.
3. The distal point used to create energy in the area is LI 4. Do not stimulate this point at length during the first few months of pregnancy and at menstruation time. An alternate point of P 8 can be used in these cases.
4. The proximal point is TH 15, which is situated on the trapezius muscle halfway between the tip of the shoulder and the spine. Balance energy between this point and LI 4. This particular balance represents a very powerful energy balance, and is useful to create relaxation in the whole of the arm, not just the lateral

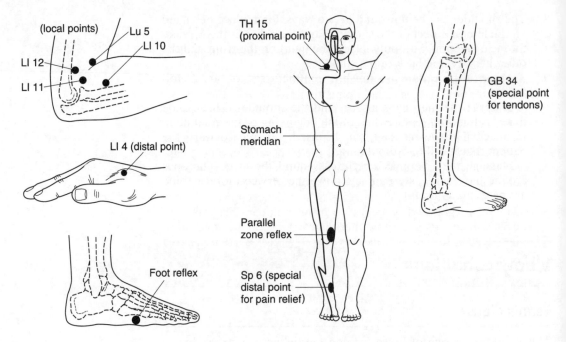

Figure 7.7   Points used in the treatment of tennis elbow.

aspect of the elbow. Often the patient will say that the whole arm feels heavy, almost leaden.

5.   Next, balance between the lesion (often LI 11) and LI 4. As with many of the conditions treated, this balance will easily and fairly quickly change the emphasis required so as to produce very rapid healing in the tissues. It offers a good deal of pain relief (almost numbness) in the area.

6.   The lesion is now balanced with the reflex points. There is a useful one on the lateral aspect of the foot. A tender point will also be found on the medial aspect of the knee, which represents the parallel zone reflex. This can be quite a useful balance. Balancing with the parallel point on the other elbow can also be profitable.

7.   The special point for tendinous lesions, GB 34, should be stimulated and then balanced with the lesion. If the lesion is more of a muscular one, the special point is Li 3. There is also a special distal pain relief point situated approximately at Sp 6. It isn't always exactly on Sp 6, and depends whereabouts on the elbow the actual lesion is, but there will always be a tender point!

8.   There are two ways to unwind the lesion; first, with the hands lateral and medial to the elbow joint, and secondly, with the hands anterior and posterior to it.

Golfer's elbow

Golfer's elbow is the inflammation of the tendons of the wrist flexors at the medial epicondyle. It is caused by putting too much strain on an extended and laterally strained elbow with the hand and wrist in tension. It is common amongst golfers, practitioners of some of the more vigorous martial arts and also physiotherapists.

Treatment

1. The associated meridian of the wrist flexors is the stomach. This should be stroked, together with the meridians that lie close to the lesion – i.e. the small intestine and the heart.
2. There are only two meridian points that are close to the lesion – Si 8 and Ht 3 (Figure 7.8). Si 8 is situated in the posterior aspect of the cubital joint, in a depression between the olecronon of the ulna and the tip of the medial epicondyle of the humerus. Ht 3 is situated between the medial end of the transverse cubital crease and the medial epicondyle of the humerus when the elbow is bent. These two points need to be stimulated.
3. The distal point to create energy is Si 3. This is a powerful point in its own right, and is ideal as a distal point in this condition because it lies on the same meridian as one of the main local points and is also on the same vertical zone. Si 3 is situated at the

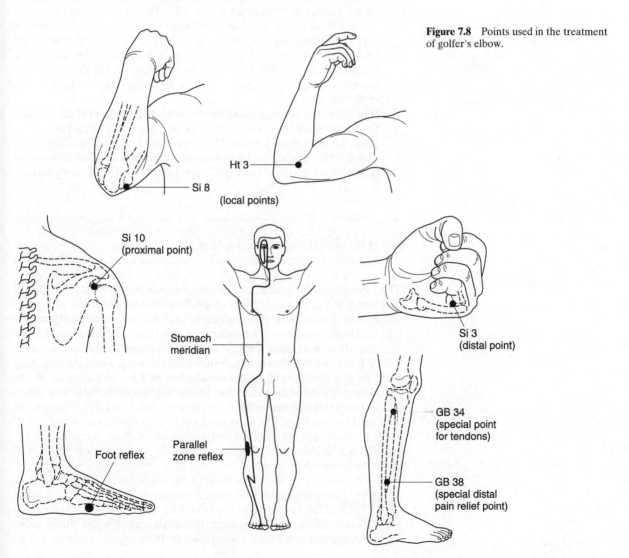

Figure 7.8   Points used in the treatment of golfer's elbow.

Ht 3

Si 8

(local points)

Si 10
(proximal point)

Stomach
meridian

Si 3
(distal point)

Foot reflex

Parallel
zone reflex

GB 34
(special point
for tendons)

GB 38
(special distal
pain relief point)

end of the transverse crease proximal to the fifth metacarpo-phalangeal joint when the hand is half-clenched. Si 3 is not usually a very tender point, and care should be taken that it is actually being stimulated!!

4. The proximal point for this lesion is at Si 10, which is one of the points on the posterior aspect of the shoulder joint used in the treatment of shoulder conditions. It is situated directly above the axillary fold, on the lower border of the scapular spine. Hold these points for about 2 minutes in order to create a flow of energy through the lesion.

5. The lesion is now balanced with Si 2. Hold this balance until a change of energy emphasis is made. This sometimes takes up to 2–3 minutes. A relief in tension around the medial aspect of the elbow should now be felt.

6. The main reflex points for the medial aspect of the elbow are the parallel point on the other elbow, the foot reflex and the parallel zone reflex point, which is situated on the lateral aspect of the knee. Therapists often get confused with this! The lateral aspect of the elbow is reflected on the medial aspect of the knee and *vice versa*. The easy way to remember it is that the thumb is reflected with the great toe and the little finger with the little toe. If the hand is placed on the foot, the forearm has already been pronated thus giving the anatomical positioning that indicates the reflected area.

7. Stimulate the special point for tendons, GB 34, and then balance this point with the lesion. There is also a special distal pain relief point approximately at GB 38 (depending on where the lesion is).

8. Finally, the lesion can be unwound by placing one hand over the lesion and the other over the lateral aspect of the elbow joint.

Carpal tunnel syndrome

This condition represents one of the most crippling of all the repetitive strain syndromes, and is extremely common amongst sedentary workers and manual workers alike. It seems to be particularly prevalent in those who use a keyboard all day long. The symptoms are inflammation and pain on the anterior compartment of the wrist. There is often parasthesia associated with the pain, and also radiating pain up the arm. These symptoms are caused by entrapment of the neurovascular bundle under the flexor retinaculum. There is often classic medial nerve parasthesia of the first three and a half fingers, as well as the dorsal tips. Patients tend to drop things for no reason, and there is often coldness in the hand. Please *check the cervical region* for any cervical lesion before assuming that all the symptoms arise from the wrist – they may not!!

Treatment

1. The meridians that pass over the wrist, namely the heart, pericardium and lung meridians, need to be stroked in the direction

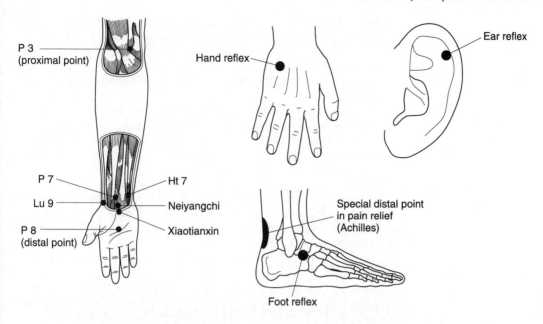

Figure 7.9 Points used in the treatment of carpal tunnel syndrome.

of energy flow. There is no associated meridian for this condition using applied kinesiology philosophy.

2. There are five points that are used as local stimulating points. They are the three Yin points of the wrist, namely Lu 9, P 7 and Ht 7, plus two extra meridian points called Neiyangchi and Xiaotianxin (Figure 7.9). They are very close to each other, and often the obvious thing to do is to massage any tender point in the area – it's non-scientific, but seems to work.
3. The distal point to create energy is P 8 (in the middle of the palm). This should be stimulated for at least 2 minutes before any reasonable amount of energy is built up ready to be used. The more chronic the condition, the longer it takes to build up the energy.
4. The proximal point is P 3, which is in the middle of the elbow crease. As stated before, P 3 and P 8 are both minor chakra points and are therefore ideally suited for this condition. They are also on the same meridian and the same zone.
5. Next, balance the lesion with P 8. These two points are quite close together anatomically, and it is important that they are held for at least 3 minutes. When the lesion is very chronic and painful, it will take a very long time to balance these two points, but perseverance is needed. In time there will be a change of emphasis, and the wrist joint will suddenly become less painful and more comfortable. There will also be a lot of heat produced at the wrist, as well as tingling and heat being produced all the way up the arm to the neck.
6. Now balance the lesion with the reflected points of the wrist. There is an excellent one on the ear, as well as others on the foot and hand (Figure 7.9). A more than useful one is the other wrist crease.
7. There is a special distal pain relief point that is to be found on the Achilles tendon. The therapist can either place individual fingers

on the wrist and Achilles to create a balance, or place the whole of the hand on each. It is a matter of individual taste and comfort. As with the seeming irregularity with the elbow reflexes, the anterior wrist is reflected on the posterior aspect of the ankle (Achilles) and the dorsum of the hand is reflected on the front of the ankle joint.

8. Unwinding is often done with just two or three fingers placed over the lesion and the same number of fingers of the other hand on the back of the wrist. It is also useful to mobilize the cervical spine in order to release tension at the roots of the median and ulnar nerves.

The use of clinical acupressure really comes into its own in the treatment of this condition. The therapist will find that there is much more rapid relief of pain and return to function than when using orthodox treatments.

Symphysis pubis inflammation

The symphysis pubis is a fibrous joint, so it has very little natural movement. There is slightly more movement in females than in males to allow for expansion during pregnancy and childbirth. The symphysis pubis is often injured during pelvic crush injuries that occur in road traffic accidents or during a heavy compression force, as in parachuting. The joint can simply be inflamed due to inflammatory congestion of the underlying pelvic organs or to repetitive trauma in sports that place a lot of pressure on the area, such as triple jumping. In the author's opinion, though, in order to have a 'weakness' in the area of the symphysis pubis, there has to be a previous weakness within the whole pelvic mechanism. This could often be a lumbo-sacral condition or sacro-iliac inflammation.

Treatment

1. As the area to be treated is in a 'delicate' region of the body, it is not necessary to perform any meridian massage, although some short strokes along the kidney meridian would be an advantage.
2. The local points are shown in Figure 7.10. They are Con 2, which is situated in the midline just above the symphysis pubis, extra meridian point Longmen, which is situated in the midline at the lower end of the joint, and Ki 11, situated bilaterally just half a cun lateral to Con 2. Great care should be taken in massaging these points. They can be *very* tender. It is often the case that, although there may be an underlying chronic condition, the actual area is usually very painful and inflamed and, of course, very tender. Therefore it would be excellent just to place the fingers on the points and allow them to 'drain' or sedate, as if it were a totally acute condition.
3. The distal point to create energy is Ki 6. This point, which is situated just below the medial malleolus, is a specific point for pain

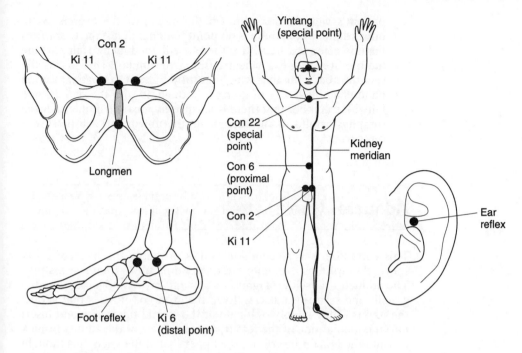

Figure 7.10 Points used in the treatment of symphysis pubis inflammation.

relief for the anterior pelvis and groin area. It lies in the same vertical zone as the symphysis pubis, and is therefore ideally situated. Ki 6 will be quite tender if the joint is sore.

4. The proximal point is Con 6, 2 cun below the umbilicus. In severe and chronic cases, Ki 6 and Con 6 need to be stimulated quite heavily at the same time before the points are energy balanced. When this occurs, there is a definite relaxation of the localized tissues and the patient will often comment that a 'warm glow' is being produced in the pubic area.

5. Now that Ch'i energy has been allowed to flow through the lesion, the next stage is to treat the inflammation. The painful point above or below the pubis is held with the finger of one hand and energy balanced with Ki 6. This should be held for anything up to 5 minutes. The pubic area will become less and less painful as these two points are held.

6. The reflex points for the symphysis pubis are the foot reflex and the ear. The ear, especially in this condition, can prove very useful.

7. There are two special points that can be used in this condition, namely Yintang (Extra 1) and Con 22. They are both situated in the mid-line of the body, hence in the same vertical zone, and they are both chakra points. Con 22, at the sternal notch, is also the parallel region to the symphysis. These particular balances can prove very effective. It would be good if the hold could be prolonged in order to produce a change of emphasis.

8. Unwinding of the joint takes place with one hand placed over the symphysis pubis and the other hand placed over the sacrum. This is also a well-known hold in cranio-sacral therapy. The patient can be either supine or side lying. When the patient is lying supine, the hand that is underneath the sacrum has to take the

patient's weight, and although the object of the exercise is to unwind the lesion, there is no point in doing that if the therapist's hand is being crushed!! It is therefore a good idea to support the lumbar spine with a wheat cushion or similar. This leaves the sacrum free, without having the full weight of the patient on the hand. The ideal way of doing it, though, is with the patient side lying. Remember that there is hardly any movement in either the symphysis pubis or the sacrum, so the unwinding will be slow – but sure!!

Adductor (groin) strain

This condition is very common and is probably the bane of every sports therapist, as it is quite often very difficult to treat successfully. The adductor muscles (magnus, longus and brevis), together with the gracilis and sartorius muscles, form the group of muscles that adduct the femur. They mainly originate at the ischial tuberosity and insert into the medial side of the femur, although part of the adductor magnus and the gracilis insert into the upper end of the knee. It is thought that, in primitive man, the medial ligament of the knee was part of the adductor magnus. Groin strain occurs either as a one-off injury or as a repetitive strain syndrome. It is common with sudden stretching of the adductors, such as slipping on ice. It is also common in racket sports players, who lunge a lot, but it is probably most common in footballers and rugby players who slip on muddy pitches. There is pain and inflammation either right into the ischial tuberosity insertion or along the belly of the muscles as far as halfway down the medial aspect of the thigh.

Treatment

1. The associated meridian for the adductors is the pericardium. This needs to be stroked three or four times in the direction of energy flow. It is also an advantage to stroke the kidney, liver and spleen meridians, as they lie locally to the area.
2. There are no specific local points shown in Figure 7.11. This is because there is a plethora of meridian, non-meridian (extra) and reflex points in the area. It is simply enough to massage the whole of the area in a firm yet reassuring manner. This area of the body is very tender in people with no problems, and of course it is in a *very* 'delicate' area. Please be careful not to be too firm with the acupressure; also, if treating a member of the opposite sex, it is diplomatic to have a chaperone in the room!
3. Energy is created at Ki 6, which is the point that was used in inflammation of the symphysis pubis and one that is used in pain relief in the lower pelvic and groin areas. As before, this point needs to be stimulated for 2–3 minutes until a build-up of energy is felt under the finger.
4. The proximal point is at Ki 16. This point is situated just lateral to the umbilicus. It is a suitable point because it lies in the same zone

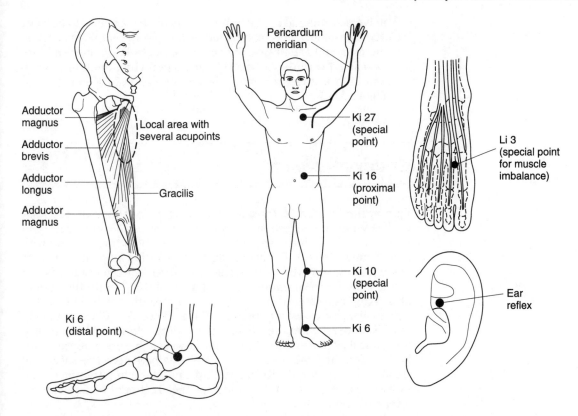

Figure 7.11   Points used in the treatment of groin strain.

as the groin, and it also lies on the kidney meridian – the same as the distal point. The points Ki 6 and Ki 16 need to be balanced so that Ch'i can flow through the lesion. This may not be easy to achieve in some cases, either because of congestion in the area or because of the patient's inability to relax! Reassuring words are needed here!!

5. The patient must now indicate the most painful point. This is sometimes difficult to do in an area where it is all very tender. The most tender point should be held and balanced with Ki 6. This part of the procedure is often the most effective, and it is at this stage that patients start to relax, both their modesty and in terms of pain relief.

6. The tender point is now balanced with the reflexes associated with the groin. There is a useful point in the ear, but the best one is the parallel point on the other groin.

7. There are three special points. Stimulate Li 3, which is the special point for any kind of muscle imbalance. It should now be balanced with the lesion. Another special point is at Ki 27, which is situated under the medial aspect of the clavicle at the very proximal end of the kidney meridian. This balancing allows relaxation to take place in the pelvis and abdominal region as well as the groin. The final special point is distal to the lesion at Ki 10. This point is situated on the medial aspect of the knee joint, very close to Li 8. It is used purely as a pain relief point.

8. The best way to unwind the groin muscles is to place one hand on the lesion area and the other hand under the patient on the sacro-iliac joint. As in the case of the symphysis pubis, there is very little

movement that takes place and the unwinding is bound to be slow.

9. The treatment can be completed by doing some gentle massage in the area and then using the acupressure holding points that are associated with the pericardium meridian. Hold the points Ki 10 and P 3 for a few seconds, followed by points Li 1 and P 9 (see Figure 5.6c).

Chronic hip pain

Pain in the hip can be caused by osteoarthritic changes in the joint itself, by pelvic congestion and inflammation to the sacro-iliac and lumbo-sacral junction (referred pain), or by inflammation with malalignment of the femoral head due to an injury to the knee or ankle joint. Conservative physiotherapy treatment usually consists of gentle exercise, heat, mobilizing and deep massage, with the patient also taking anti-inflammatory drugs. Acupuncture has been found to help in arthritic cases with the use of heated needles. Because the hip joint is so deep within the pelvis, it presents a formidable challenge for clinical acupressure. There can, however, be great rewards for both patient and therapist if there is a little patience. The successful treatment of a chronically painful hip can take many treatment sessions. This, of course, holds good for the treatment of any chronic joint condition.

Treatment

1. The gall bladder meridian is the only meridian to pass through the hip joint, so this is the ideal one to energize by stroking with the flow of energy – i.e. downwards from the head towards the foot. However, it would also be an advantage to stroke all the other meridians that lie close to the hip joint, namely the stomach, liver, kidney and bladder.

2. There are several meridian and non-meridian acupressure points that lie close to the hip joint and can be used in the early stages of a treatment, regardless of where the pain lies. It is always useful to massage each point for a few seconds. This not only improves the energy flow (blood and lymph) to the area, but is also useful as a diagnostic tool when it comes to finding the most painful point to be used later in the treatment. On the anterior aspect, the points are Li 12, Sp 12 and Sp 13. On the lateral aspect are points GB 29 together with three non-meridian points – Jiankua, Kuanjiu and Qiangkua. The posterior part of the hip joint gives us GB 30 and Zuogu (Figure 7.12). As there are several more non-meridian points and reflex points that become tender when there is pain and congestion around the joint, it would not be a bad idea to find a painful point and massage it. No harm can be done by using this simplistic approach; in fact, just the opposite – the more points that are energized, the better.

3. The best distal point to use in order to create energy is Ki 1 (on the sole of the foot). This point represents the most powerful

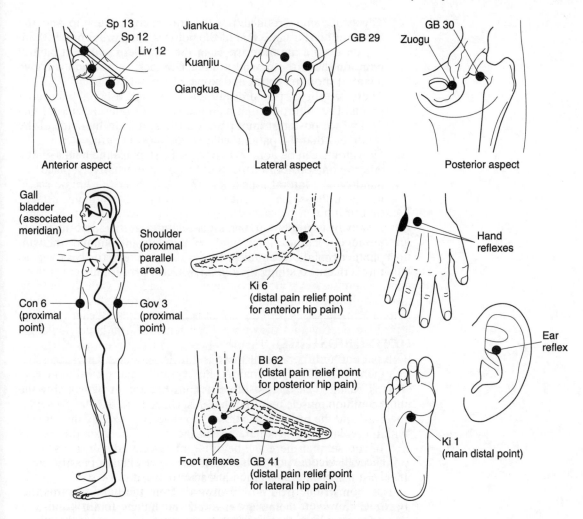

Figure 7.12 Points used in the treatment of chronic hip pain.

distal point that will be effective in relieving pain in the hip joint and surrounding soft tissue. As with each and every chronic condition, the distal point needs to be stimulated for up to 3 minutes before enough workable Ch'i is produced.

4. There are two proximal points. Con 6 (2 cun below the umbilicus) is used for anterior hip pain and Gov 3 (L4–5) is used for lateral and posterior hip pain. One or possibly both points are balanced with Ki 1 to ensure energy flow through the joint. It is worth bearing in mind again that the practitioner must not will anything to happen and that it is the patient's own energy system that is being used for healing, that concentration is maintained on the joint being treated. In other words, when treating the hip – think hip.

5. The next stage is to find the most painful point (there may be more than one) and balance this point with Ki 1. It goes without saying that, if there is more than one painful point in the hip area, then each has to be balanced with Ki 1 in turn.

6. The main reflexes for the hip are the ones in the ear, foot and hand. Please note that there are two reflexes on the hand and foot, depending on which part of the hip has the most discomfort.

The other main reflected areas are the opposite hip and the shoulder on the same side of the body as the painful hip. If there is pain on the anterior aspect of the hip there will be a painful point on the anterior aspect of the shoulder; lateral pain will give a lateral shoulder reflex and so on.

7. There are three special distal points that are used as pain relief points. For antero-medial pain use Ki 6, for lateral pain use GB 41, and for posterior joint pain use Bl 62. It is at this stage of the treatment that the patient will feel the most benefit.

8. Unwinding can be done in two ways. First, place the hands on the anterior and posterior aspects of the joint; alternatively, place one hand on the lateral aspect and the other over the lumbo-sacral junction. Please be patient in this part of the treatment, it takes time!!

9. Finally, it is good to do some general massage around the whole hip region that will improve the blood flow and enhance the lymphatic circulation. The best type is connective tissue massage, as this is the most stimulative of all massage procedures.

Torn hamstring

This is included in the list of conditions because it is probably the most common muscle tear that therapists have to treat. The principles involved and the order of treatment, however, are exactly the same as with muscular tears anywhere else in the body. The main differences are, of course, that there will be different associated meridians, distal points and proximal points, but these can be worked out easily by the therapist using the information already provided.

The hamstring group of muscles often tears in the middle, between the semi-membranosus and the biceps femoris muscles. There are several degrees of tear and subsequent trauma; these range from a slight pull or overstretch through to interstitial rupture of a muscle. The latter could require surgery. The most common type of hamstring tear, however, is a partial rupture of the belly of one of the muscles intrastitially. This means that there is initial bleeding into the muscle with resultant pain and stiffness, followed by slow consolidation and healing. Without treatment there is usually a telltale 'lump' of scar tissue to be found in an old torn hamstring. This represents a potential weakness. As with all acute muscle tears, do not do any acupressure for the first 24–36 hours following trauma. The bleeding has to be allowed to stop, aided by ice, compression and elevation of the leg, before treatment can commence. The ideal time to commence acupressure treatment following trauma is 72 hours later.

The hamstring is usually torn because of sudden tension in the muscle. This is caused by a number of factors, including old scar tissue within the muscle, misalignment of the pelvis due to an old injury that causes imbalance in the muscle, over-striding caused by bad coaching, or an old inversion sprain of the ankle. Acupressure treatment serves two purposes:

- To initially ease pain, discomfort and swelling and to bring about resolution
- To rebalance the cause of the condition – i.e. to realign the pelvis or ankle. This will obviously make it less likely for the muscle to pull in the future.

Treatment

1. The associated meridian is the large intestine meridian. In cases of acute lesions where there is much swelling and pain, the meridian should be stroked against the flow of energy (nose to hand). In all cases of chronic tears, the meridian should be stroked in the direction of energy flow. This should be done four or five times. In cases of chronic lesions, it is also good to massage the bladder meridian downwards.
2. No local points have been indicated in Figure 7.13. This is because, in this instance, it is unimportant. In acute injury, place the finger onto the lesion, gradually getting deeper and deeper

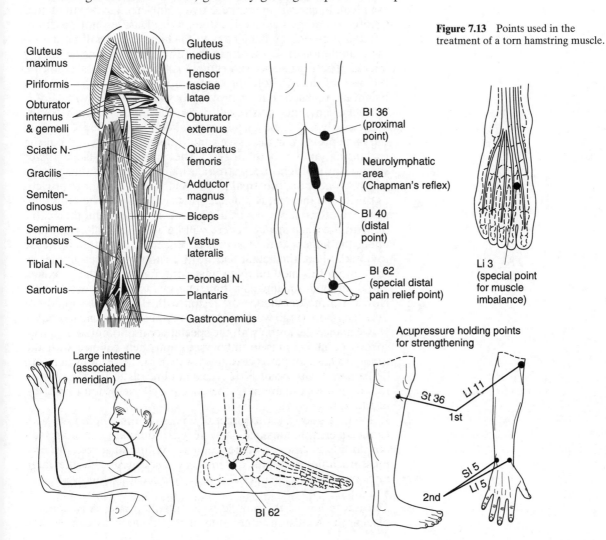

Figure 7.13 Points used in the treatment of a torn hamstring muscle.

into the tissues as the patient allows (see Chapter 4 for a description of the technique). This will bring out quite a lot of heat and inflammation. In cases of chronic injury it is simply sufficient to massage around the lesion, concentrating especially on the distal part of it. This will help tracking of exudate fluid and consolidation of the tissues. It is also pertinent at this stage to massage the associated Chapman's reflex for the hamstring, which is situated on the medial aspect of the thigh. This is a very tender area and care should be taken, although the massage has to be stimulating in order to be of any use!!

3. The distal point is Bl 40, which is situated in the middle of the popliteal fossa. It is a very powerful and influential point, and should be stimulated for about 3 minutes in the case of chronic tears. Where there is an acute tear, Bl 40 should be stimulated just for a few seconds.

4. The proximal point is Bl 36, which is situated in the middle of the gluteal fold. Both the proximal point and the distal point are on the same meridian and also lie on the same vertical zone, so they are ideal. In chronic tears, these two points need to be stimulated before an energy balance is attempted. Please do not be disappointed if an energy balance is not achieved; this will be due to the granulation or scar tissue in the lesion area causing an energy 'block'. The next stage is very important. Using massage oil on the back of the leg, hold the two points (Bl 36 and Bl 40) until a balance is reached (but, as previously stated, do not worry if it is not achieved), then push gently into the tissues at both points. Very slowly move the finger from Bl 40 towards Bl 36, keeping the same pressure in the tissues and (hopefully) keeping a pulsing (balancing) under both fingers. The proximally placed finger should stay still. This deep stroke is maintained right through the lesion towards the proximal point. As the distal finger approaches the lesion, the energy balance will usually stop. When this happens, wait for a few seconds until it recommences and then carry on with the deep stroke. There will be a definite different 'feel' under the fingers as the lesion is approached, and often it is easy to detect where the actual tear is, no matter how deep in the tissues, using this method. Now place the fingers on the proximal and distal points again. This time energy flow will be easily felt.

5. Now it is time to balance the lesion with Bl 40. This should not take long due to the work that has previously been carried out.

6. Now balance the lesion with the special points. Stimulate Li 3 (the special point for muscle imbalance) and then balance with the lesion. In cases of pain (virtually always), the lesion now needs to be balanced with point Bl 62. This hold needs to be done for up to 3 minutes until an energy balance is achieved (don't time it – just let it happen!!).

7. It is now a good idea to generally massage the whole area with connective tissue massage or some such stimulating massage (do *not* do this in cases of acute lesions). At this stage use the acupressure holding points for muscles associated with the large intestine. Hold St 36 and LI 11 for a few seconds, followed by LI 5 and Si 5.

8. The unwinding of the muscle is essential!! It is usually done by placing the hands on either side of the lesion. This can be very

comforting for the patient. The unwinding procedure will pave the way for attempting to treat the cause of the lesion, whatever it is. If it is caused by over-striding, it may be a job for the coach. If it is caused by pelvic imbalance, this is put right by easing the sacro-iliac joints and providing a stable leg length (see Chapter 8). In the case of sprained ankle aetiology, place one hand over the lesion and the other hand over the lateral aspect of the ankle. Balancing and gentle unwinding should now take place. Frequently the ankle joint has to be mechanically aligned by whatever manipulative procedure is normally used.

Do not expect instant miracles with this procedure. The patient (athlete) will, however, experience much more comfort in the area. Stretching exercises can be taught and carried out in subsequent treatment sessions as the lesion improves.

Knee conditions

Medial ligament lesion

As anyone who has suffered from this condition will know, this lesion can be one of the most painful conditions that therapists have to treat. It is caused by a sudden forced lateral strain at the knee joint. Examples of the aetiology are kicking a heavy ball with the instep, a 50/50 tackle in football, slipping in mud, or over-lunging (doing the splits) with subsequent adductor magnus muscle strain. As shown in Figure 7.14, there are two parts to this ligament – deep and superficial fibres – which have different distal attachments. The superficial fibres were once thought to be an extension of the adductor magnus muscle. The medial ligament can be just 'tweaked' (superficial fibres), partially torn (causing pain and instability to the knee joint) or totally ruptured. The latter necessitates surgery. Acupressure is very useful in the treatment of a pulled or partial tear, and also in rehabilitation following surgery.

Treatment

1. Stroke the three Yin meridians of the leg (spleen, kidney and liver) in the direction of energy flow – i.e. from the foot upwards.
2. There are four local points, although there are several minor trigger points in the area. The points are Sp 9, Li 8, Ki 10 and a non-meridian point called Liaoliao, which is situated at the proximal end of the ligament. These points should be stimulated when there is a chronic lesion and sedated in acute conditions.
3. The distal point to create energy is Ki 6, which is situated just inferior to the medial malleolus of the ankle joint. As previously explained, this point is specific for pain relief in the groin and down the medial aspect of the leg. It therefore serves as both a distal point to create energy and as a distal pain relief point.

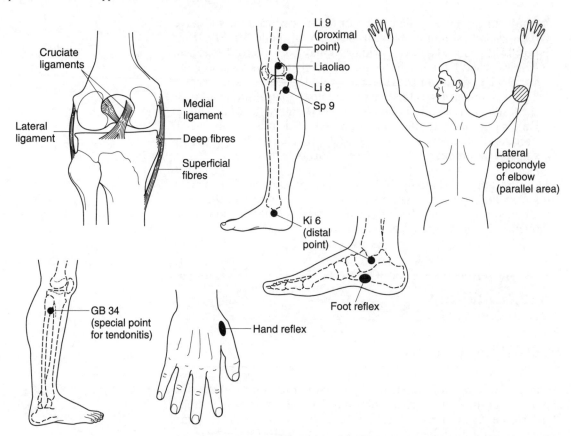

Figure 7.14   Points used in the treatment of medial ligament lesion.

4. The proximal point is Li 9, which is situated 4 cun superior to the medial epicondyle of the femur between the vastus medialis and sartorius muscles. Ch'i energy flows through the lesion when the distal and proximal points are balanced, although it is not always possible to create a balance when the ligament is badly injured.

5. The next stage is to balance between the lesion and Ki 6. The painful part of the medial ligament usually lies directly over the joint margin. This hold, for a period of over 2 minutes, should produce a change of emphasis, thus giving quite a lot of pain relief in the area.

6. Next, the lesion is balanced to the associated reflex points. The best and most effective one is the lateral aspect of the elbow (parallel area). There will always be a tender area to be found around the lateral aspect of the elbow in all cases of medial knee pain. The foot reflex can prove a useful pain relief point, as can the hand. Don't forget to balance the lesion with the other medial ligament on the opposite knee.

7. Now stimulate GB 34 (special point for tendinitis) and then balance this point with the lesion.

8. The medial ligament is unwound by placing one hand over the lesion and the other hand over the lateral aspect of the knee. Not much actual movement is created underneath the hands, but the whole area will start to feel more comfortable to the patient afterwards. Don't forget to teach the patient some gentle exercises to strengthen the quadriceps and adductors.

Chronic knee pain

Chronic knee pain can be caused by osteoarthritic changes, ligamentous lesions, chronic bursitis to any part of the joint and subluxation of the superior tibio-fibular joint, as well as many other named conditions. The knee joint represents probably the most complicated joint in the body. It does not have very congruent surfaces, and is subject to a great deal of (physical) stress-related torsion. Acupressure is a real alternative to the tried and tested methods of treatment of heat, mobilizing and exercises. These other modalities can still be performed when doing acupressure. As stated before, never forget any of the other skills that have taken years to learn and perfect.

Treatment

1. As in all cases of chronic joint lesions, all the meridians that flow through the joint should be stroked initially. Therefore, the three Yin meridians of spleen, liver and kidney should be stroked from the foot upwards and the three Yang meridians of stomach, gall bladder and bladder should be stroked downwards towards the foot.
2. As shown in Figure 7.15, there are several meridian and non-meridian local points at the front and back of the joint. During

Figure 7.15 Points used in the treatment of chronic knee conditions.

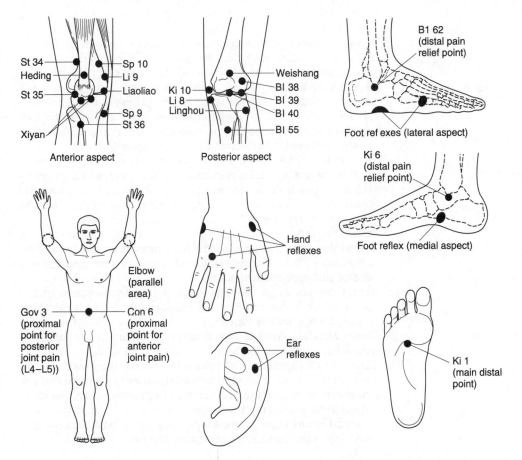

the initial part of the treatment, it does not matter where the lesion or pain is. It is beneficial to stimulate *all* the local points regardless of the lesion site. Spend about 10 seconds on each point. The patient will soon let you know which ones are tender! The points that seem to be the most effective are St 35 (situated in the depression just below the patella, lateral to the quadriceps tendon), Ki 10 and Li 8 (mentioned together as they are very close to each other at the very medial aspect of the knee), Bl 40 (situated in the middle of the popliteal fossa), Bl 39 (1 cun lateral to Bl 40), Liaoliao (situated on the prominence of the medial condyle of the femur at the proximal end of the medial ligament) and two points with the same name – Xiyan (these are bilateral points situated below the patella in the hollow either side of the quadriceps tendon). Xiyan is often called the 'eyes of the knee' and these two points are extremely effective in pre-patellar and infra-patellar pain and swelling. All the other points should be stimulated, but the ones mentioned appear to be most effective.

3. The general distal point for all chronic knee conditions is Ki 1 (sole of the foot). As with any chronic joint pain, this point has to be stimulated for quite a long time in order to create enough Ch'i to be used in the treatment.

4. There are two proximal points, depending on the site of most discomfort. If the lesion is on the anterior aspect of the knee, the proximal point is Con 6 (2 cun below the umbilicus). If the lesion is more postero-lateral, the proximal point is Gov 3 (between L4 and L5 in the mid-line). These points need to be stimulated before attempting an energy balance through the joint. In the section about treating a chronic hip joint it was mentioned that the practitioner should think 'hip' when trying to balance the patient's Ch'i through that joint. This time, it helps to think 'knee'. It tends to focus the attention on the job in hand; after all, the hands are spread well apart, with one on the sole of the foot and the other on the abdomen or lower back. It is not a question of using the power of the mind in order to heal!!

5. The hardest procedure is to find the most tender point. As with the hip, there may be several, and each should now be balanced with Ki 1. It will soon become clear which ones are reacting and which are not. The easier it is to create a balance, the less the point needs treatment; the harder it is to balance in the early stages, the more it needs treatment. Remember that in chronic lesions the energy is deep within the joint, and it has to become superficial before changes occur. So don't be disappointed if a balance does not occur readily.

6. Next, the lesion is balanced with the main reflected points on the rest of the body. There are three reflex points on the hand, three on the foot and two in the ear, again depending where the joint is mostly affected. An excellent balance of energy can be achieved with the parallel area of the elbow as well as the other knee.

7. There are two special distal pain relief points; the much used Ki 6 and Bl 62. These are to be found just below the medial and lateral malleolii. Ki 6 is used for antero-medial knee pain and Bl 62 is used for postero-lateral pain.

8. The joint is unwound in two ways. First, place both hands either side of the knee front and back; secondly, place the hands medial

and lateral to the joint. Be prepared to keep the hands *in situ* for about 5 minutes. This part of the treatment is always the most beneficial in chronic joint treatment, and is the one that gives most comfort to the patient.

9. The treatment session can be finished with long or short strokes of deep massage around the joint and some mobilizing. Please remember that it is very beneficial to mobilize the patella and the head of the fibula.

Post-knee surgery quadriceps strengthening

This short section has been added as a result of several requests from physiotherapists who find that attempting to strengthen the quadriceps following a meniscectomy or other knee surgery can prove very difficult. Whilst the post-surgical bandages are *in situ* it is obviously impossible to perform any local acupressure; however, do not forget that the remainder of the treatment regimen can be carried out. If it is impossible to place the fingers onto the lesion because of bandage restriction, the option is to use the same point on the opposite knee. There are two special procedures that can be carried out at the end of the painful knee treatment previously described:

- Using the stretch reflex on the scalp
- Using the acupressure holding points that are associated with the quadriceps.

The stretch reflex on the skull is situated on the forehead just above point Extra 1. It lies between the stretch reflex for the sternocleido-mastoid muscle and the, temporo-mandibular joint. Place the fingers either side of the reflex and gently stretch the fingers away from each other. Hold this for about 2 minutes (see Figure 3.14).

The quadriceps is associated with the small intestine when using the applied kinesiology procedure of acupressure holding points. First, hold points GB 41 and Si 3 for a few seconds, followed by points Bl 66 and Si 2 (see Figure 5.6b). There will be an immediate 'take' by the quadriceps, indicating the flow of Ch'i to the muscle. From that moment on, the physiotherapist will find that a quadriceps contraction will be facilitated, leading to a straight leg raise and other exercises being performed successfully!!

Shin splints

Shin splints is a composite term that describes pain, inflammation and swelling along the tibia. There are two main types; anterior tibial compartment syndrome, which is inflammation of the tibialis anterior, and medial tibial compartment syndrome, which is inflammation of the tibialis posterior. These are the main muscles that are affected, although others often come into the equation. This condition occurs in athletes, and is often due to changing training or performance routine – for example, training on soft ground as opposed to roads, suddenly increasing the tempo of training or changing the shoes. The latter is the most common. When the author served with the Royal Marines, the vigorous training in new boots that had no 'give' in them seemed to be the main cause of inflammation in the tibialis posterior and pain along the medial aspect of the shin. The toes attempt to grip and cannot, thus producing a tension force further up the muscle. Anterior compartment syndrome is really a condition of repetitive strain. Both types of shin splints can be very painful, often cripplingly so, and can ruin the careers of budding athletes if not treated early and correctly. The use of acupressure (and correct diagnosis) has revolutionized the author's treatment of this condition.

Treatment

1. The tibialis anterior and the tibialis posterior are both associated with the bladder meridian. Stroke this meridian in the direction of the energy flow, i.e. from the eye to the little toe.
2. No local points have been indicated in Figure 7.16 because, in both these painful conditions, the whole area is tender. It is therefore advantageous in chronic conditions initially to try some deep

Figure 7.16   Points used in the treatment of shin splints.

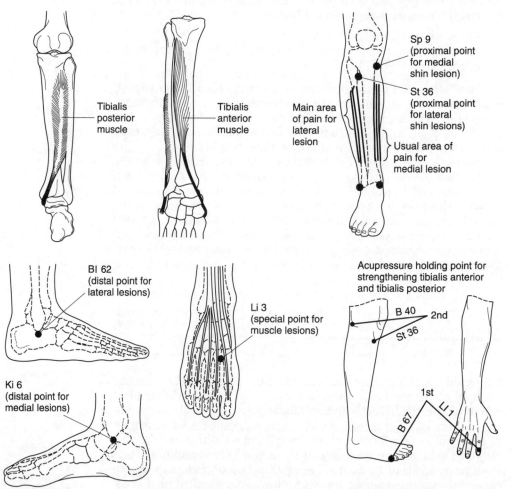

massage strokes (to the patient's tolerance) vertically down the lesion area. This type of massage will immediately produce hyperaemia and thus start the healing process. Experience has shown that the most painful area on the tibialis anterior is at the middle to upper aspect of the tibia, whereas the painful area on the tibialis posterior (medial aspect of the shin) is at the lower third of the tibia (around the Sp 6 area).

3. There are two distal points, depending on the location of the lesion. For lateral lesions it is Bl 62, and for medial lesions it is Ki 6. These two points need to be stimulated. In sub-acute conditions (acutely painful, but chronic in length of time) not much stimulation will be needed in order to create enough Ch'i to use for treatment.

4. Again, there are two proximal points. For lateral lesions it is St 36, and for medial lesions it is Sp 9. These two points need to be gently stimulated and then balanced, each with its respective distal point, depending on the lesion being treated. This procedure creates a good deal of comfort in the area. When a balance of energy has been achieved (not always possible if the lesion is very chronic), it is time to perform some deep controlled massage strokes from the proximal towards the distal point in a manner similar to that described in the treatment of a torn hamstring. This has to be done with the patient's pain tolerance in mind. Do not continue if it becomes too painful. This part of the treatment may be performed after balancing with the distal point, which also will help with pain relief.

5. Next, the lesion (most painful part) is balanced with the distal point. It is often the case that the most painful part covers more than one finger's breadth; if this is so, use two or possibly three fingers at the lesion site.

6. The lesion area can now be balanced with the reflected area. There is only one of note – on the other shin!! There does not seem to be a parallel area on the arm, and experience has shown that the foot, hand and ear reflexes are not effective.

7. The only special point is Li 3, which is used in any muscular condition. This point will always exhibit varying degrees of tenderness, depending on the acuteness of the lesion. At this point it is desirable to use the acupressure holding points that are designed to strengthen muscles associated with the bladder meridian. First hold Bl 40 and St 36 for a few seconds, followed by Bl 67 and LI 1.

8. To unwind the lesion, it is simply enough to place the hands proximal and distal to the lesion site on the muscle. It is also an advantage to place one hand proximal to the lesion and the other hand over the medial or lateral aspect of the ankle joint. Mobilizing the whole foot, including the metatarsals, will also be helpful.

Achilles tendinitis and pain

Achilles tendinitis is yet another of those soft tissue conditions that can be very difficult to treat successfully without continued recurrence. The condition varies in severity from simple inflammation of the sheath caused by faulty footwear with the Achilles tab rubbing on the tendon, through several stages of tendon inflammation and partial rupture to, finally, total rupture. The latter often happens as a result of sudden over-stretching when the tendon is cold (i.e. not warmed up). A typical example would be at a father–son school cricket match, with the very unfit father making a dash for a quick single off the first ball – the screams are heard in the next village!! Total rupture obviously needs surgical intervention. The following treatment rationale can be used in post-operative situations as well.

Treatment

1. The associated meridian for the gastrocnemius and soleus muscles is the triple heater meridian. This should be stroked three or four times in the direction of energy flow, i.e. from the hand to the face.
2. There are several local points that can be used to stimulate (or sedate in the case of acute tendinitis) in the initial stages of the treatment. The points on the medial side of the Achilles are all on the kidney meridian, and those on the lateral side are on the bladder meridian. There are two extra meridian points called Genping and Quanshengzu, which are on the tendon itself. Genping is situated in the middle of the Achilles on a line exactly between the inferior aspect of the medial and lateral malleolii, and Quanshengzu is situated in the middle of the tendon at the superior border of the calcaneus (Figure 7.17).
3. The distal point to create energy is Ki 1 (sole of foot). This will need to be stimulated for 2–3 minutes in chronic cases.
4. The proximal point is Bl 40, which is situated in the middle of the popliteal fossa. There should be no problem in balancing Ch'i between Bl 40 and Ki 1. It is a common balance procedure that is used in the treatment of low back pain and sciatica (see Chapter 8).
5. Find the most painful point or area on or around the Achilles tendon and balance it with Ki 1. The most painful point is commonly at the narrowest part of the tendon, which corresponds to point Genping. This point can also be balanced with Bl 62 and Ki 6, depending on which side of the tendon is the most painful.
6. The main reflex points for the Achilles tendon is at the palmar aspect of the wrist joint. It is best to balance on the wrist of the same side of the body. A tender point will always be found at the wrist with this condition.
7. Stimulate GB 34 (special point in tendinitis) and balance it with the painful point. Next use the acupressure holding points associated with the triple heater meridian. This means holding points GB 41 and TH 3 for a few seconds, followed by points Bl 66 and TH 2. These points will energize the gastrocnemius and soleus muscles.
8. The Achilles is unwound by having the patient lying prone with the ankle supported but overhanging the end of the couch. Place one hand in the lower bulk of the gastrocnemius muscle and the other hand on the posterior aspect of the heel. Unwinding will take place fairly rapidly, depending on the chronicity of the condition.

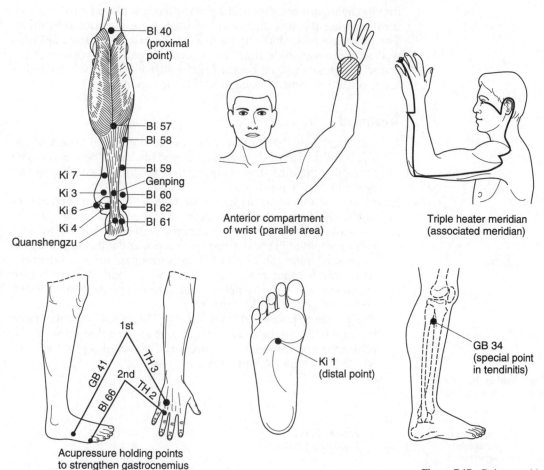

Figure 7.17   Points used in the treatment of Achilles tendinitis and pain.

9. Finally, it is beneficial to do some deep massage either side of the tendon (as pain permits).

Lateral sprain of the ankle joint

This condition represents one of the most common injuries that therapists have to deal with. The initial treatment of an acutely sprained ankle at the hospital accident department is often woefully inadequate. It is one of those injuries where attention to detail in the first-aid stage of treatment can make so much difference to the future well-being of the person. The stability of the ankle is so vitally important for having a correctly aligned leg, spine and cranium. There have been hundreds of cases presented in the author's clinic of headaches and cervical spine imbalance that have been caused by a sprained ankle, maybe 20 years previously, that wasn't treated correctly initially. As well as giving cold application and elevation, it is imperative that the ligaments are supported and the ankle is placed into eversion, thus allowing the torn ligaments to heal in the functional position. The following procedure can be used in the case of an acute ankle as well as a chronic ankle that has become perpetually weak over the years. The points will be handled differently in each case; sedated in acute conditions and stimulated in chronic conditions.

Treatment

1. The meridians that run over or near to the lateral aspect of the ankle are the stomach, gall bladder and bladder. These need to be stroked in the direction of energy flow for chronic conditions and against in acute ones.
2. Most of the local points lie on the bladder meridian. The exception is GB 40, which lies just in front of the lateral malleolus.
3. The distal point used to create energy is Bl 66 (Figure 7.18). This point is situated in the depression anterior and inferior to the fifth metatarsal bone. This point will also stimulate urine production, so be careful that the patient has had a 'comfort stop' before treatment! Do not attempt to stimulate this point if there is any cystitis or similar bladder inflammation.
4. The proximal point is at point GB 34. This point is the ideal one because it lies on the same vertical zone as the ankle sprain and it is also the special point for tendinitis. Balance this point with Bl 66 – don't forget to think 'ankle'.

Figure 7.18   Points used in the treatment of lateral sprain of ankle joint.

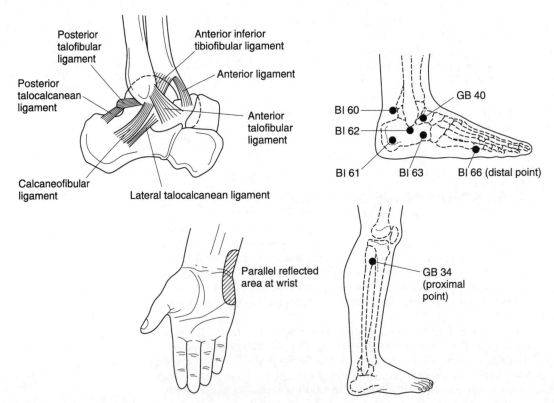

5. The painful point or area is now supported energically by balancing it with the distal point. In cases of chronic lesions, this could take anything up to 4 minutes or so.
6. There are two main reflected areas for the lateral aspect of the ankle; the opposite ankle and the ulnar border of the wrist joint. These two areas should be balanced for at least 2 minutes each. The wrist balancing is especially important. In chronic conditions it is also an advantage to balance the ankle area with the lumbar spine, especially if a weakness in the ankle has brought about lumbar spine pain.
7. It is now beneficial to balance again between GB 34 and Bl 66. This reinforces what has been achieved so far, and also strengthens the bladder and gall bladder meridian so as to have a stronger ligament and thus a more stable ankle joint. Prevention is better than cure!!
8. The area is unwound by placing one hand over the lateral aspect and the other hand over the medial aspect of the ankle joint.
9. Finally, some stimulating or connective tissue massage in short strokes around the ankle will help the healing process.

Metatarsalgia and foot pain

There are many causes of this painful condition. The metatarsals can be acutely painful due to ill-fitting shoes, walking too far on hard ground (repetitive strain) or injury or accident. A more serious and chronic form of this condition, often named Morton's metatarsalgia, is where there is nerve inflammation between the metatarsal bones. This can be caused by a displaced metatarsal head, or is a chronic form of an acute metatarsalgia that was not treated. It really is not good enough when patients are fobbed off by the GP with a prescription for anti-inflammatory drugs in the vain hope that somehow a metatarsal head will miraculously adjust itself and ease the pain. Treating mechanical conditions with drugs is about as silly as visiting an osteopath with chickenpox!!

Treatment

1. All the meridians that pass over the foot may need to be stimulated – in the direction of flow in chronic conditions and against the flow in acute conditions.
2. Although there are several non-meridian points, as well as Ki 1, situated on the plantar aspect of the foot, it is only necessary to stimulate (chronic) or sedate (acute) the painful points. These are shown in Figure 7.19. The patient will always advise where the painful point lies!
3. The distal points are the tsing or nail points. They are the end points of the liver, spleen, stomach, gall bladder and bladder meridians. One of these should be stimulated, depending on which toe extension the condition lies.
4. The proximal point is at Bl 40 in the middle of the popliteal fossa.

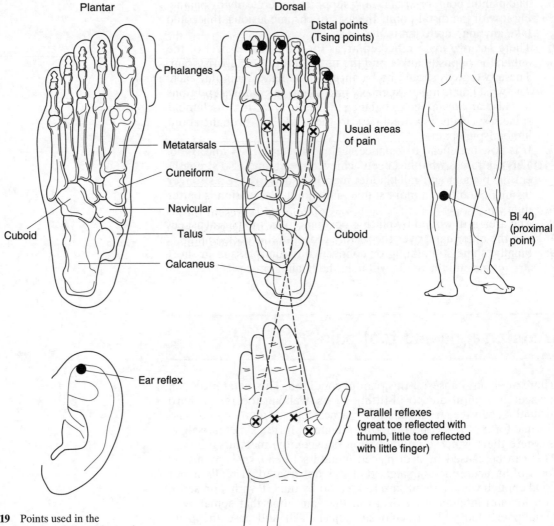

Figure 7.19 Points used in the treatment of metatarsalgia and foot pain.

This point should be stimulated and then balanced with the appropriate tsing point, thus allowing a flow of energy through the lesion (think 'foot').

5. Now find the most tender point and balance it with the selected tsing point.

6. The reflected area that is most used in metatarsalgia is on the palmar aspect of the hand. Remember that the great toe is reflected with the thumb, the little toe is reflected with the little finger, etc. A painful point will always exist at the appropriate point of the hand in all cases of foot pain. Time should be taken to achieve a balance between these two points. There should be a shift of emphasis if possible. There is also a very useful reflex point in the ear that can be used in acute conditions.

7. It is at this stage that an adjustment of the metatarsal head can be carried out (if this is the cause of the problem). The soft tissue sit-

uation around the lesion should be much more flexible and comfortable after the previous treatment, and a simple adjustment should not present the therapist with too much difficulty or the patient with too much discomfort.

8. The foot is unwound by placing one hand on top of the foot and the other hand underneath. A further unwinding procedure is to place the hands underneath the foot and at the back of the knee.

Summary

As stated previously, the 19 conditions mentioned represent only a fraction of what therapists treat in their everyday work. Regardless of the condition, though, the 'batting order' and the procedure remain the same in each and every case. Practice makes perfect!!

8

Treatment of spinal conditions

Analysis and assessment

There are literally scores of different spinal conditions. Each gives a different set of signs and symptoms, and it would be impossible to cover all of them in this chapter – that would require a whole book. It is possible, however, to break down the symptomatology into what is easily definable – acute and chronic. Within reason, apart from some neurological conditions, it does not matter what the definitive diagnosis is – the treatment, using clinical acupressure, is the same!! Doctors and therapists often get bogged down in attempting to find a definitive diagnosis, when all the time it isn't really necessary. Of course, professional therapists have to use judgement and discernment with regard to conditions that fall outside their scope of clinical practice and expertise; if in doubt, do not tackle the problem but put the patient in the hands of someone who can cope with the given situation.

Acute spinal conditions

Acute conditions of any kind all give the same symptoms of pain (local and/or referred), muscle spasm, inflammation and localized deformity. If not treated correctly during the first 48 hours after the lesion occurs, there will always be a 'knock on' effect of pain and acute deformity elsewhere in the spine (Lovett brother), and possibly pain and stiffness in a peripheral joint.

Almost immediately after an acute lesion occurs, the reflected point or pathway will be tender. These (as has been discussed at length elsewhere) are situated in the hand, foot, ear, temple, skull, and other parts of the spine. Palpation of these reflected points (reflexes) will indicate exactly where the lesion is, if this is not apparent on localized palpation of the vertebral column. Examples of acute spinal lesions include:

- Muscle tears (to varying degrees) of the deep intravertebral muscles. These produce pain, localized inflammation and swelling, but rarely localized deformity.
- Ligamentous tears (to varying degrees) of the intervertebral ligaments. These produce pain, spasm, inflammation and localized deformity, resulting in the apophyseal joint becoming subluxed or hyper-stretched.
- Nerve root inflammation. This is caused by sudden over-stretch or lateral disc protrusion and produces very acute pain (local and radiating), localized muscle spasm and inflammation. This can result in neuritis of the whole length of the inflamed nerve (e.g. in sciatica).
- Centralized disc protrusions. These cause excruciating localized and referred pain, spasm and inflammation. Complete rest and anti-inflammatory medication (allopathic, homoeopathic or herbal) is the only initial treatment for this condition, but acupressure can help tremendously after the first 48 hours.

It is often the case that an acute spinal lesion happens as a result of a chronic (long-lasting) spinal weakness that may have been caused as a result of a fall or other trauma as a child. The damage is done in infancy, and the person spends many years compensating for their underlying weakness. Eventually, during some activity or another (it does not have to be strenuous), the original weakness will give rise to acute symptomatology.

Chronic spinal conditions

Examples of chronic spinal conditions include:

- Muscular lesions. These may be the result of a series of microtraumas or because the spine attempts to compensate for an old postural imbalance. Microtraumas to the spine can be caused by repeated falling as a child or teenager either onto the coccyx region or onto the side (off a horse or fence, slipping on ice, in the playground at school etc.). Old postural imbalances are caused (obviously) by faulty posture as a child or teenager – slouching, sitting incorrectly for many hours at a time, insufficient exercise or trying to compensate for being tall. There is usually local and distal pain, muscle spasm, lymphatic circulation inflammation or congestion, and sometimes formation of fibrositic nodules within the muscles themselves. This is called fibrositis or fibromyalgia as a generalized set of symptoms, or lumbago if occurring in the lumbar spine. It seems that many doctors and therapists dismiss lumbago as a trivial or non-diagnosed condition. It is very real!!

- Ligamentous lesions. These are caused by old postural imbalances as above, or as a result of repetitive over-stretching of ligaments. Shortening and thickening of the interspinous ligaments occurs, causing fixations of two or more vertebrae. There is diffuse pain and spasm, plus localized and distal deformity.
- Chronic conditions following acute disc lesions of the cervical and lumbar vertebrae (rarely thoracic) where there has been inadequate or no treatment during the acute phase. There is multiple muscular spasm, ligamentous shortening and thickening, often fibrositic nodule formation and sluggish blood and lymphatic circulation. There is a great deal of pain that is both local to the original lesion and also diffuses out to affect other areas of the spine, as well as peripheral areas.
- Congenital deformities such as scoliosis, kyphosis, lordosis and others. These do not always give resultant symptoms in later life, but often do. There is sometimes a case here for gentle palliative treatment that eases pain and spasm, thus making everyday functional tasks easier to perform. Vigorous therapy and surgical intervention can result in worse long-term prospects of quality of life at the expense of a more mobile spine!
- Conditions that occur as a result of surgical intervention, e.g. spinal fusion, laminectomy, discectomy etc. Clinical acupressure works very effectively in this ever-increasing category of patients. The therapist has to realize, though, that the results achievable are only as good as the surgical intervention will allow.

Treatment of acute spinal conditions

In any acute spinal condition or lesion there is a similar 'batting order' of treatment to that used in acute peripheral joint conditions. As with soft tissue lesions anywhere in the body, it is not always to the patient's advantage to treat acute lesions until at least 24 hours after the injury or trauma. Before that, it is best to have the patient put an ice pack (or bag of frozen peas) wrapped in a towel directly onto the lesion.

Order of treatment

1. Palpate the area gently and find out where the lesion is. Massage the local points around the lesion. At this early stage, it could be an advantage to place the finger(s) onto the painful site to try and release the inflammation (as previously described).
2. Create energy at the most convenient distal point. This point is always on the spine.
3. Find a suitable proximal point (either on the spine or the skull, but it is always a point on the governor meridian) and balance Ch'i between the proximal and distal points, thus allowing energy to flow through the lesion.

4. Balance the lesion with the distal point.
5. Balance the lesion with suitable reflex points or powerful points that are nearby. These could be on the same vertical zone as the lesion, or the best pain relief points – e.g. LI 4 for cervical pain or Bl 62 for lumbar pain.
6. If there is a subluxation that needs adjustment, now is the moment to do this – very gently, by utilizing the patient's body's mechanics and not by brute strength. A simple subluxation of an apophyseal joint will reduce very easily once the muscle tension has been reduced by previous work on the lesion.
7. Finally, if the cause of the lesion has been eased (e.g. spasm, subluxation, haematoma etc.), the lesion can now be unwound. This is usually carried out by placing the pad of the middle finger on the painful point and the pad of the other middle finger on exactly the same point on the opposite side of the vertebra. It usually takes a couple of minutes to ascertain a change of emphasis under the fingers. It is then that slow and gentle unwinding will take place, normally with lateral and rotational movements. As with unwinding of peripheral lesions, it is either the therapist's fingers or the patient that moves as the unwinding takes place. It is usually the former, although if your patient expresses the wish to move the neck or lower back, then allow this to happen. Finally, it would be wise to mobilize the adjacent vertebrae as well as gently mobilizing the offending one. Home exercises should also be taught.

Acute cervical lesions

In order to treat an acute lesion successfully, it is not always necessary to have a pinpoint accurate diagnosis. How many professional therapists have had patients referred from the GP or specialist with a particular diagnosis only to discover that the problem is quite a different one? Therapists have to learn to think on their feet, and quite often a diagnosis will be forthcoming once the process of treatment has commenced.

Treatment

1. Accurately identify the site of the lesion by gentle palpation around the area. The patient should be lying down and comfortable, preferably in the supine position with the head supported on a small wheat cushion or similar. Place a pillow under the knees so as to minimize lower spinal discomfort. Previous questioning and analysis will have shown if there is a disc lesion or nerve root lesion with referred pain or parasthesia. If this is the case, it is important that the arm with the referred pain should be supported with a pillow or wheat cushion. It is hopeless to attempt to gain muscle relaxation in the area if the shoulder and arm are screaming with pain due to faulty positioning. Once the patient is comfortable and the lesion has been located, proceed gently to massage the acupuncture points (meridian, non-meridian or trigger) adjacent to the lesion. Figure 8.1 shows the location of many of the more important local points. This diagram is not exhaustive,

Figure 8.1 Local points used in the treatment of cervical lesions.

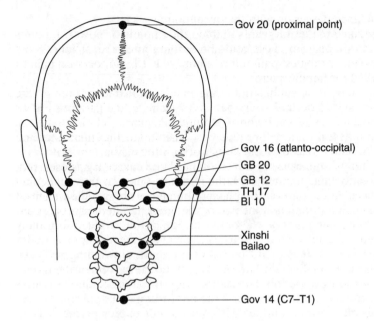

and if there are other points in the area that are tender, then massage them!! Now place the pad of the middle finger into the lesion or painful area, very slowly increasing the amount of pressure to the patient's tolerance. This procedure could take a couple of minutes. If the patient finds this uncomfortable, do not do it but proceed to the next stage.

2. For lesions occurring between the sub-occipital area and C6, the distal point is Gov 14, which is situated between C7 and T1 in the interspinous space. For C7 lesions, the best distal point is Gov 10, which is situated between T6 and T7. Massage this point for up to half a minute, or until there is an obvious energy build-up under the finger.

3. The best proximal point is Gov 20. This point is situated on the top of the skull, exactly halfway between the base of the skull and the eyebrows in a direct line between the anterior aspect of each ear. It is a very powerful point, being the physical aspect of the crown chakra. Balance between Gov 20 and Gov 14 (or Gov 10) in order to create an energy flow between these two and thus through the lesion. It does not matter if the lesion is slightly off-centre (it usually is).

4. Now place one finger on the lesion site and the same finger of the other hand on the distal point. Dwell for a couple of minutes on this balance, until a change of emphasis occurs. By now there should be much lessening of pain and tension in the area.

5. Now balance the lesion with the many surrounding points. These may include:

    A point on the same vertical zone – if the lesion is a subluxed apophyseal joint and is (obviously) slightly away from the midline, the best vertical zone reflex is Bl 11, situated under the transverse process of T1 (see Figure 8.2). This can be a surprisingly comfortable and gratifying balance in that it brings quite a lot of comfort and ease to the area.

A distal pain relief point – the best one is LI 4, situated on the first interosseous muscle between the thumb and forefinger. Use the LI 4 that is on the same side of the body as the lesion.

Another useful point – for example, LI 15, which is situated at the point of the shoulder underneath the acromion head; TH17, which is situated in a groove under the inferior aspect of the ear; or points under the base of the occiput. GB 20, GB 12 and Bl 10 are also useful points to be used in balancing.

6. There will be sufficient release of the supporting ligaments and muscles to now perform an adjustment of the vertebra (if this is the cause of the lesion). If a rotational subluxation has occurred, the procedure is to support the head and gently rotate it, keeping the middle finger on the upper subluxed vertebra. The weight of the patient's head should be all that is needed to produce a spontaneous release. There should be no thrust technique used; allow body mechanics to do the work.

7. Bring the patient's head back to the normal position and place the finger pads of the middle fingers on either side of the lesion. This will allow unwinding of the local tissues. The adjacent vertebrae may be mobilized (Maitland or similar), and finally the problem vertebra itself can be moved gently in a postero-antero direction.

Further treatment may be necessary 2–3 days later, and inner range neck extension exercises should be taught in order to start the process of strengthening the supporting muscles.

Acute thoracic (dorsal) lesions

It is rare to experience a disc lesion in the thoracic spine, but the most common lesion is an acute flare-up of an old postural condition, which gives muscle spasm. Other lesions include acute fibrositis, rib facet subluxation and apophyseal joint subluxation, as well as acute muscular tension of the trapezius muscle due to stress and tension. The main acupuncture points associated with this area of the spine are those on the 'inner' bladder line from Bl 11 to Bl 21. These are situated 1.5 cun lateral to the spinous process in the gap between the transverse processes. Before acupressure treatment commences, try some gentle massage in the area to release the superficial muscle spasm. It may not be possible, though, due to pain and spasm.

Treatment

1. Palpate the area to locate the lesion. Now massage all acupuncture points adjacent to the lesion. This may not be possible due to pain. Proceed to the next stage if it cannot be done.

2. The best distal points to create energy are Gov 10, situated between the spinous processes of T6 and T7 and used in upper thoracic lesions, and Gov 6, situated between the spinous processes of T12 and L1 and used in lower thoracic lesions (Figure 8.2). The relevant point should be stimulated for up to half a minute, or until enough energy is created for treatment – it does not take long in acute conditions.

Figure 8.2 Some points used in the treatment of acute and chronic spinal conditions.

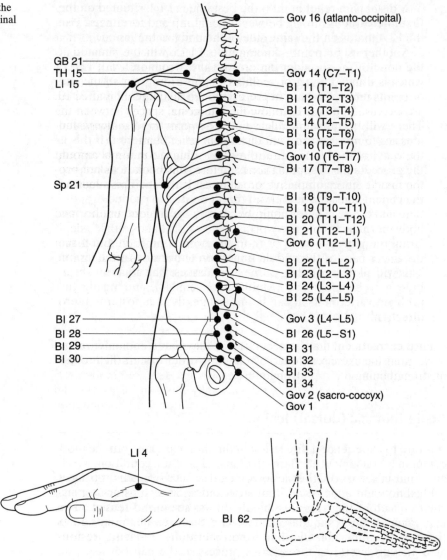

3. The ideal proximal point is Gov 14, which is situated between the spinous processes of C7 and T1. This should now be balanced with either Gov 10 or Gov 6 to allow energy to flow through the lesion.
4. Find the lesion (the most painful point) and balance it with the distal point. Hold this balance until a change of emphasis occurs.
5. Next, balance the lesion with other suitable points. These could lie on the same vertical zone (superior or inferior to the lesion), or use points GB 21 and TH 15 in upper thoracic lesions. These two points will always be very tender in upper thoracic and lower cervical lesions as they are situated in the trapezius muscle, which nearly always exhibits spasm in local lesions. The most effective point to use in the treatment of thoracic spine lesions is Sp 21. This point is situated in the sixth intercostal space in the mid-axillary

line. Use the point that is on the same side as the lesion. It makes an excellent pain relief point. Although Sp 21 is the main pain relief point, there are many other related non-meridian points that are equally effective, depending on the lesion. If the diagnosis is one of rib facet subluxation or apophyseal subluxation (with or without joint rotation or scoliosis), choose the pain relief point according to the transverse process/rib articulation that is affected. Wherever the lesion is, follow the intercostal space (between the ribs) down to the mid-axillary line. The point there is always tender, and makes an excellent distal pain relief point.

6. Now adjust the lesion (if required) by using the minimal amount of force. As has been mentioned before, this book does not propose to teach manipulative procedures. If the therapist does not feel competent to manipulate – don't do it!

7. Unwind the area if necessary by placing the fingers superior and inferior to the lesion, or by placing the whole hands either side. It is then important that the thoracic spine is mobilized and that shoulder, cervical and thoracic mobilizing exercises are taught to take the patient through to the next treatment.

Acute lumbar spine lesions

Acute lumbar spine lesions are amongst the most commonly treated conditions in a therapist's surgery. The only other condition that may be more common is the chronic lumbar lesion! As stated in the preface to this chapter, acute lesions come in all shapes and sizes, and can vary enormously as to degree and type of pain, spasm, inflammation etc.

Treatment

1. Locate the lesion and the possible cause. Massage the area if possible (with oil), and also fingertip massage the surrounding acupoints. Although Figure 8.2 only shows the points situated on the bladder meridian, there are several more tender points to be found, both meridian and non-meridian, in acute lesions. Massage whatever is tender – gently!!

2. The distal point for lesions of L1 and L2 is Gov 3, which is situated between the spinous processes of L4 and L5. The distal point for lesions of L3–L5 is Gov 2, which is situated between the sacrum and coccyx (Figure 8.2). Massage the distal point for about 30 seconds to create some energy in the area, although in an acute lumbar spine there is usually Yang Ch'i overflowing in abundance.

3. The proximal point used is Gov 6, which is situated between T12 and L1. Balance between the proximal and distal points to allow energy to flow through the lesion.

4. Now place the finger on the actual lesion (most painful point) and balance it with Gov 2. Hold this balance for at least 3 minutes, or until a shift of emphasis has taken place. By now the lumbar area should be feeling less tense and sore.

5. Next, balance the lesion with associated distal points. These may include:

A point (or points) on the same vertical zone. This could be superior to the lesion at the cervico-thoracic junction, as in Bl 11, or inferior to the lesion, using one or more of the many bladder points that are situated on the sacrum.

A distal pain relief point. The most effective distal pain relief point is Bl 62, which is situated just underneath the lateral malleolus. Other distal points used are Bl 40, which is in the middle of popliteal fossa, and Li 8, which is on the medial aspect of the knee.

Reflex points on the foot and hand. These are very effective in treating the acute lumbar spine, and will be fully discussed in the later section on chronic spine conditions.

6. The lumbar spine should now be much more comfortable and in a better position for any kind of adjustment to be carried out without undue discomfort. If the condition warrants it, then do some mobilizations plus further gentle massage to the area.

7. Unwind the lesion by placing one hand over the sacrum and the other hand over the lower thoracic region – i.e. either side of the lesion. In acute syndromes the process of unwinding does not take very long but can be quite dramatic to witness, both for the practitioner and the patient. This aspect of the treatment is very effective. It is essential that home exercises are taught, preferably those that will strengthen the lumbar spine but will not provoke any further trauma and subsequent inflammation.

Sacro-iliac pain and inflammation

The sacro-iliac joint can be acutely traumatized in several different ways. The most common one is repetitive strain of the joint due to constant bending with twisting. Another common reason is a sudden compression strain on the joint, usually caused by walking along and suddenly stepping down further than the previous stride. The sacro-iliac joint can also become inflamed after falling badly from a horse or high object, or slipping on ice or mud and landing heavily on the back, or inflammation may be due to a chronic condition. There can be just localized pain, or radiating pain down the sciatic nerve.

Treatment

1. Pain and spasm can be present for the whole length of the palpable section of the sacro-iliac joint or in just one small section of it. Where the pain is diffuse, finger pads of at least three fingers are needed for palpation and subsequent treatment. Try to massage the area if this can be tolerated by the patient. Also massage the surrounding acupoints. These can be the bladder meridian points that lie over the sacro-iliac joint (Bl 26–30), or those bladder meridian points that lie in the sacral foramen (Bl 31–34) (Figure 8.2). Try to keep the fingers still over the painful area to release the excess inflammation; this could take up to 2 minutes.

2. The best distal point to create energy is Gov 2, which is situated at the sacro-coccygeal junction. Stimulate this point for up to 1 minute.

3. The proximal point is Gov 3, which is situated between L4 and

L5. Although it is a mid-line point, it has far more power and therefore is more effective. Balance Ch'i between the proximal and distal points in order to ease the tension in the area.

4. Now place the finger(s) onto the painful part of the joint and balance with Gov 2. This hold should last as long as it takes for a change of emphasis to occur.

5. Balance the lesion with the following points:

    Effective points on the same vertical zone. Inferiorly this is Li 8, which is on the medial aspect of the knee joint, and superiorly it is any point on the inner bladder line – possibly the best points are Bl 11 and Bl 23.

    A distal pain relief point. The best distal pain relief point is Bl 62, which is found just underneath the lateral malleolus. Be aware that initially this balance could produce more discomfort, but further holding will give the anaesthetic treatment that is needed. Further points will be discussed in the section on chronic sacro-iliac joint conditions.

6. If the underlying condition is one of a joint subluxation, an adjustment should now be done. The patient is usually positioned in side lying for the adjustment; if this is the case, take care not to inflame the tissues again.

7. Unwind the sacro-iliac joint by placing one hand over the sacrum and the other hand on the side of the hip. Alternatively, the patient can lie supine and be made comfortable with cushions to support the lumbar spine and knees. The therapist sits at the side of the couch, and places one hand underneath the sacrum, allowing the patient's weight to settle onto the hand (this may take a few seconds). The other arm is placed on the upper aspect of the pelvis with the forearm resting on the nearby anterior superior iliac spine and the fingers on the other anterior superior iliac spine. This is a very popular treatment technique in cranio-sacral therapy, and can be used for sacral malalignment as well as for sacro-iliac syndromes.

Sciatica

Sciatica is the inflammation of the sciatic nerve, and ranks as one of the most painful conditions that therapists have to deal with. It is mentioned in this section of acute conditions, even though it is usually caused by an acute flare-up of an established condition in the lumbo-sacral spine. The procedure described below can be used in chronic conditions as well. Sciatica can radiate into the buttock, to the back of the knee or all down the leg to the outside of the ankle. It can be an extremely disabling condition.

Treatment

1. Pain is often very diffuse, and it is difficult sometimes to have a single point that exhibits more discomfort than another one. Usually the best local point is Bl 28, which is situated on the sacro-iliac joint to the lateral side of the second sacral foramen (Figure 8.2). Massage the points that are adjacent to this point if the patient can tolerate it.

2. The distal point to create energy is Ki 1, which is situated on the sole of the foot. This has been found to be the best distal point that encompasses the complexities of this condition. Stimulate this point for up to 2 minutes.
3. The best proximal point is Gov 3, which is situated between the spinous processes of L4 and L5. Balance between this point and Ki 1.
4. Now place the pad of the middle finger onto the most painful point and balance it with Ki 1. This balance may last for up to 3 minutes. Try and reach a shift of emphasis under the fingers, although it may not always be possible due to the extreme discomfort of the patient.
5. There are several reflex points to be used:
   The foot reflex is very useful. This is situated around the heel. It is not just a single point, but rather a band that encompasses the heel. Slowly work along the whole length of the reflected area whilst keeping the finger of the other hand on the local point.
   The main distal pain relief points are Bl 40, which is situated in the middle of the popliteal fossa, Bl 62, which is situated just below the lateral malleolus, and Bl 66, which is situated near the end of the little toe on the lateral border. With the finger of one hand placed on the local point, place the same finger of the other hand on each point in turn, starting with Bl 40, until a balance of energy is created. This procedure may take up to 5 minutes, but the pain relief that can be achieved is sometimes quite remarkable.
6. It should now be possible to perform mobilizations of the lower lumbar spine and also of the sacro-iliac joint. This will help release the tension that exists in the great nerve. There is no unwinding procedure with this condition. It also helps to stretch the psoas major muscle and take pressure off the piriformis and gluteus maximus muscles using pressure techniques.

Because of the degree of discomfort that exists with this condition (remember that the sciatic nerve at its broadest is over 2 cms wide), the therapist will not provide instant relief in just one treatment session. However, experience has shown that this approach of using clinical acupressure is superior to any other technique, including acupuncture. As has been stated before, sciatica can have a complicated aetiology; it is not always caused by a prolapsed intervertebral disc!! It can be caused by several other spinal anomalies, and sometimes by a sluggish and heavy large bowel or chronic cystitis. Ask the patient questions!!

Coccydinia (inflamed coccyx)

Anyone who knowingly pulls a chair away as someone is about to sit on it, even as a prank, can have no idea what painful torment is in store for the victim of this mischievous and cruel act. In coccydinia, the coccyx can be subluxed both ways (95 per cent of the time anteriorly), dislocated, or the supporting ligaments can be over-stretched and torn. It is an extremely painful condition, and ranks alongside sciatica on the pain scale. It is very difficult for the patient to sit down with any degree of comfort, even on a soft chair. If the acute version of this condition is not treated successfully, the patient will develop further musculo-skeletal changes of the pelvis and lumbar spine, which in time can affect the thoracic and cervical spine. Because of the delicate anatomical positioning of this lesion and subsequent treatment procedure, it is best to have a chaperone in the room. Do not take chances!!!

Treatment

1. With the patient comfortably lying prone, gently palpate around the region of the lower sacrum and the coccyx to ascertain the specific lesion. In the author's experience, the most common lesion is an antero-lateral subuxation that over-stretches and tears the cornual ligaments, which in turn affect the musculature of the perineum. Care should be taken in palpation, and please do not attempt to treat this condition with no previous experience! There is no need to massage the surrounding points; the lesion will be too painful. The local points are Gov 1 and Gov 2 (Figure 8.2).
2. The best distal point is Ki 1 (described in the treatment of sciatica). This point will need to be stimulated for up to 1 minute.
3. The proximal point is Gov 3, which is situated between L4 and L5. Balance Ch'i between the proximal and distal points.
4. Now gently place the fingertip of the middle finger onto the lesion and balance it with Ki 1.
5. Keeping the finger *in situ* on the lesion, place the middle finger of the other hand on the reflex point of the foot. This is situated on the medial aspect of the inner border, by the heel, and represents a very powerful point. Dwell a couple of minutes on this balance. The lesion can now be balanced with the main distal pain relief point of the lower spine, Bl 62. It is also beneficial to balance the lesion with Gov 16, which is at the atlanto-occiput. As will be described in the treatment of chronic conditions, balancing with the associated Lovett brother vertebra can be useful.
6. If the lesion is simply a partial ligament tear with no bony misalignment, the treatment is now concluded, save mobilizing the coccyx and sacrum. If there has been some misalignment, now is the time to adjust the coccyx, by whatever means the therapist is familiar with. If in doubt – don't do it!! More damage can be caused by faulty manipulations than existed in the first place.
7. When the adjustment has been made, it is beneficial to massage the area as well as the lumbo-sacral region. Finish the treatment with gentle massage of the coccyx reflex points on the feet.

Treatment of chronic spinal conditions

Many of the treatment procedures mentioned above can be utilized in the treatment of chronic conditions. A chronic condition is one that was originally acute and has been allowed to become chronic, either because of poor treatment or no treatment at all. Chronic conditions can still be very painful but, because of the length of time that the patient has suffered from the lesion, there will have been several other musculo-skeletal changes that have occurred since the initial trauma. The human frame has a marvellous way of attempting to heal itself by creating all manner of compensations such as muscle spasms, ligamentous torsions and joint misalignments. In the treatment of chronic spinal conditions, not only is it necessary to ease the patient's pain, muscle spasm and inflammation, but it is also essential to treat the cause of the imbalance. This can be achieved by utilizing the many different acupoints (meridian, non-meridian and reflex) that are associated with the area being treated. In this way, the lesion is supported energically. Once the initial assessment and analysis has been done, the first treatment can be carried out using the order of treatment outlined below. The second and subsequent treatment sessions may unearth different symptoms, and it is these new symptoms that need to be treated. As treatment progresses, the symptomatology changes according to the cause of the original lesion. The patient's energy body actually 'peels back the layers of the onion' and relives the old traumas and injuries (sometimes transiently, sometimes lengthily) until the original trauma is isolated and corrected. It is only then that the patient has been truly cured of the particular musculo-skeletal condition that was presented in the first place.

Order of treatment

1. Look at and listen to the patient.
2. General assessment of the patient's posture.
3. Specific assessment and diagnosis.
4. Balance leg length differential.
5. Massage:
    locally
    bladder meridian
    neuro-lymphatic areas.
6. Stimulate distal point.
7. Balance Ch'i through the lesion by balancing the proximal and distal points.
8. Balance the lesion site with the distal point.
9. Balance the lesion site with associated reflexes:
    parallel zone (Lovett brother)
    foot
    hand
    ear
    stretch reflexes.
10. Carry out mobilization or manipulation of vertebra.
11. Unwind the area.
12. Do a final energy balance.

At first glance this list may seem inordinately long, but in practice it will take the therapist no longer to do than any other type of assessment and treatment. The main advantage of using the order outlined above as opposed to any other is that this way uses the self-healing power of the body, utilizing energy channels. In practice this is more effective and thus minimizes the number of treatments that are needed to effect a cure. The following is a breakdown of the treatment order giving details.

Look at and listen to the patient

If detailed in full, this initial consultation procedure with the patient would fill a book. However, there are a few pearls to look out for that will give the therapist a general idea of the condition. The posture of the patient on the chair whilst relating his or her symptoms can give clues as to the chronicity of the condition and if there is any internal organ involvement. If the patient sits forward on the chair with a crouched attitude, speaks slowly and is hesitant, this quite often indicates a Yin condition that is very longstanding and where there is organic and possibly emotional change. If the patient sits in a relaxed way and talks freely and clearly, this indicates a Yang state, where the spinal lesion is in isolation without any other changes.

The tone of patient's voice can be indicative of some other pathological changes as well as spinal ones. The whining or moaning voice may indicate a gall bladder or liver imbalance, with a mid-thoracic lesion being the usual spinal anomaly. The nasal voice of a patient with catarrh may indicate a lower lumbar (L4) lesion due to the involvement of the large bowel and its association with the sinuses and the difficulty in disposing of mucus and waste matter. A person who is highly strung and 'lives on their nerves' often exhibits an upper cervical lesion, usually an atlas involvement. The man with the 'beer belly' who has allowed his general posture to sag and the muscles to weaken will almost certainly have a lower lumbar lesion with a compensatory C2 or C3 lesion. The lady who is tearful and cannot tell you her story without becoming weepy usually has an upper cervical lesion combined with an upper thoracic lesion, usually T4. The heavy smoker, with or without respiratory symptoms, will have a mid-thoracic lesion. This will give the therapist an idea of what to look for, but the list, of course, is endless.

General posture assessment

It is important that the therapist assesses the patient sitting, standing, walking, and lying supine and prone. A whole picture is essential. Check especially for the various types of gross and specific scoliosis; whether one shoulder is raised or the pelvis is hitched up on one side. The therapist must always be aware that in an 'S' scoliosis there are always three lesions and sometimes four. In all cases of pelvic and sacro-iliac imbalance there are compensatory cervical imbalances (Lovett brother) and, sometimes, thoracic imbalances as well. In cases of chronic upper cervical lesions there is usually a sacro-coccygeal lesion that needs to be treated just as much as the cervical one. Ask the patient to walk backwards as well as forwards – in this way it can be seen if there is reversed sacral tilting as well as tension in the sacro-iliac joints.

Specific assessment and diagnosis

The following should be carried out with the patient lying prone:

1. Working down the spine from the upper cervical to the lower lumbar area with two fingers either side of the spine, feel slowly and gently for any spasm, heat, tension and alteration in skin texture. Spasm always indicates muscle weakness, and is nearly always associated with that particular vertebra having a side shift or rotational subluxation on the side of the spasm. In very long-standing conditions, the subluxations are usually fixations.

2. Working down from the neck to the trunk, check for obvious lesions and abnormalities that do not have associated muscle spasm due to gross inelasticity of the surrounding tissues. Finding these lesions is not always easy, and comes with experience.

3. Check for spasm, heat and tenderness in the peripheral muscles as well as in the para-vertebral ones. It has already been shown that each muscle is related to a specific spinal level, and if a muscle is in spasm or painful, then this indicates that the related vertebra is in a state of imbalance.

4. Palpate the individual vertebra with postero-anterior and lateral movements (as in Maitland mobilizing) to check the amount of movement in each individual vertebra. The patient will tell you if there is any discomfort at each level.

5. Now check the related reflected areas for tenderness. The greater the amount of tension and discomfort in the associated reflex, the more chronic the lesion and the greater the need for immediate treatment. First check the temporo-sphenoidal line on the side of the skull. The more tender the reflex, the more the vertebra needs treatment. Then check the reflexes on the foot and hand. The foot reflex is usually more tender than the hand reflex. The reflex in the ear will also be tender, but this is generally used more in treatment than analysis. It will be noticed, however, that with very long-standing conditions the reflected areas exhibit slight swelling or puffiness as well as discomfort.

By now, the therapist will be in a much better position to know exactly what needs to be achieved in order to alleviate the gross symptoms and eventually create homoeostasis. Before the main thrust of the treatment commences, there remains one more vital test; that of checking and correcting pelvic imbalance and leg length differentials.

Balancing leg length differentials

It is most important that leg lengths are as near the same length as is possible to achieve. Almost every person has a leg length differential (due to pelvic hitching) of up to 1 cm, with few or no obvious ensuing problems. It is also true that, with some patients, even a 1 cm imbalance can produce pelvic or even atlas lesions. The leg length differential is measured with the patient lying completely flat, either prone or supine, and in as straight a postural line from head to toe as possible. The differential is measured at the prominence of the tibial (medial) malleolus and *not* at the base of the heel. There is a possibility of the patient having one of six types of leg length imbalance; Types 1–3 are very common, the others are less so. The key points of the eight extraordinary meridians are used to correct imbalances. These are all well-known points (see Chapter 2), and they are shown in Figure 8.3.

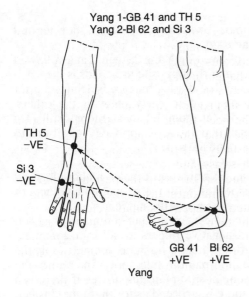

Yang 1-GB 41 and TH 5
Yang 2-Bl 62 and Si 3

TH 5
−VE

Si 3
−VE

GB 41   Bl 62
+VE   +VE

Yang

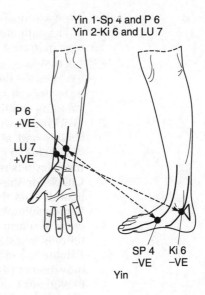

Yin 1-Sp 4 and P 6
Yin 2-Ki 6 and LU 7

P 6
+VE

LU 7
+VE

SP 4   Ki 6
−VE   −VE

Yin

Figure 8.3 Positioning of fingers on eight extraordinary meridian key points in leg length differentials.

The points are held using the pads of the middle fingers with gentle pressure until a pulsing balance is obtained – this normally takes about 20 seconds. The results are sometimes instant and remarkable. The types of leg length imbalances and their treatment are listed below.

1. Type 1 – sacral condition:
    The patient is in the prone position. Examination reveals a long leg and low buttock on the same side. When the knees are flexed, this remains the same.
    Treatment – Yin 1 (Sp 4 and P 6) on the short leg side, followed by Yin 1 reversed (change the polarity by using a different finger, e.g. the index finger) on the long leg side. If this is done correctly, there should be an immediate change in the leg length. Sometimes the patient will actually feel a 'shift' taking place in the pelvis.
2. Sacral condition with atlas involvement:
    The patient is in the prone position. Examination reveals a long leg and low buttock on the same side. When the knees are flexed, the long leg becomes short.
    Treatment – Yin 1 (Sp 4 and P 6) on the long leg side, followed by Yin 1 reversed on the short leg side.
3. Type 3 – general spinal conditions:
    The patient is in the prone position. Examination reveals a long leg and high buttock on the same side.
    Treatment – Yang 1 (GB 41 and TH 5) followed by Yang 2 (Bl 62 and Si 3), then Yin 1 (Sp 4 and P 6) followed by Yin 2 (Ki 6 and Lu 7), all on the long leg and the opposite arm. Hold each of the two points until a balance of energy is obtained, and then recheck the leg length balance. If there is no change, go on to the second hold and so on. It is not necessary to do all four holds unless it is warranted; quite often the leg differential will be balanced on the first hold. Imagine that a picture on a wall is being lined up!

4. Type 4 – low back pain:

The patient is lying supine. Examination reveals a short leg and high iliac crest on the same side.

Treatment – Yang 1 followed by Yang 2, then Yin 1 followed by Yin 2 on the short leg and the opposite arm. This is the same procedure as for Type 3 in that if a leg balance is achieved after the first hold, there is no need to carry on with the others. Furthermore, if all four holds are completed and there is still a leg length imbalance, reverse the polarity by applying Yang 1 etc. to the long leg side and the opposite arm.

5. Type 5 – sciatic nerve involvement:

Patient is lying supine. Examination reveals a short leg and high iliac crest on the same side, with the patient complaining of sciatic nerve pain along some part of the nerve.

Treatment – use positive fingers on all four command points on the painful leg side, and negative fingers on all four command points on the opposite arm. If there is no improvement, apply the negative fingers to the non-painful side foot. Then turn the patient over into the prone position and test to see if there is a Type 1–3 imbalance. If there is, proceed as for that type. Instead of using positive and negative fingers it is possible to use low gaussage biomagnets, sticking them to the points with sticky tape for up to 20 minutes. This will achieve the same result, but obviously not as quickly.

6. Type 6 – no differentials:

This may be due to a long-standing rheumatoid condition, ankylosing spondylitis or even gross osteoarthritic changes in the hips or knees – or, of course, a permanent leg length differential as a result of an impacted fracture of the femur or tibia.

Treatment – where necessary, use all four channels bilaterally with some stimulating massage.

The above procedures may, at first glance, seem to be quite complicated, but in practice they are very simple to carry out. Although treatment can have immediate results, it often has latent effects. Check leg length differentials at each visit, just to make sure the pelvis is 'seated' correctly. If the pelvis is misaligned, what hope is there for alignment further up the spine? If we correlate the pelvis to the foundations of a building, it makes sense to have strong and balanced foundations; if not, there is likelihood of the first, second and third stories (lumbar, thoracic and cervical spine) becoming misaligned. This is, of course, exactly what happens in practice.

Massage

A practical hands-on therapist need not be told of the positive advantages of massage in all its forms. Whatever the physiological and diagnostic advantages for the patient and therapist, these are often outweighed by the psychological advantages. Never underestimate the power of touch on the psyche. Patients feel more comfortable once hands are placed on them. The majority of patients are intelligent enough to appreciate that if they have a mechanical condition they need mechanical treatment, and this means 'hands on'. Various forms of electrotherapy can be applied and exercises given, but they do not feed the patient's pyschological and mechanical needs as successfully as manual therapy.

1. *Generalized soothing massage.* Initially the therapist has to feel the patient's tissues, and the patient needs to appreciate the therapist's hands. It is a two-way dialogue. General soothing massage to start any operation is so important, and it need not last long before more specific massage is carried out. It is an advantage for therapists to do a few short and long strokes of effleurage (preferably using oil) along the whole length of the patient's spine to enable them to receive information about the general condition of the patient's tissues.

2. *Local massage.* As with the treatment of acute spinal lesions, it is important to massage the local acupoints around the lesion. This involves finger-pad deep circular stimulation to all the points, making a mental note of which points are painful (the patient may even assist in the finding of a painful point by making a suitable loud noise !!). This should be done a few times, but not overdone if it is too painful. Do not live up to the reputation of being a sadist!

3. *Bladder meridian massage.* This is performed using the pads of the middle and index fingers, placed either side of the spine, and massaging with fairly heavy pressure from the neck down to the sacral area. The bladder line extends more laterally from the spine at the lumbar end than the cervical, and the spread of the fingers should accommodate this difference. In chronic spinal conditions it is necessary to improve the energic quantity in the local and distal area of the spine, and massaging the bladder meridian is one way of instigating this. When treating the lumbo-sacral spine and the sacrum *per se*, also massage along the bladder line that lies on the sacro-iliac joint and those points that lie over the sacral foramen. The use of connective tissue massage is particularly effective.

4. *Neuro-lymphatic massage.* The neuro-lymphatic areas, or Chapman's reflexes, were discussed in Chapter 3. Their use in the treatment of chronic spinal conditions is imperative. The patient has to be warned that these areas are painful!! The massaging of the ilio-tibial tract in the treatment of lumbo-sacral lesions is particularly effective. This massage is traditionally carried out without oil, but it takes a brave therapist to do connective tissue massage along the ilio-tibial tract without lubrication – it is very painful. In chronic low back and pelvic conditions, there is a good deal of lymphatic circulation obstruction and stagnation that materializes around the pelvic area and in the legs. The massaging of the neuro-lymphatic area seems to stimulate the lymphatic drainage of the local area and its associated vertebra(e).

The majority of the following procedures have been discussed in the treatment of acute lesions. There are, however, some additions. When treating chronic conditions, the therapist has to make use of every kind of reflex and associated area in order to support the local symptomatic area.

Stimulating the distal point

Having prepared the ground, so to speak, it is now that the real treatment begins. The distal point is usually a point on the spine, i.e. a governor acupoint, with the exception of coccydinia (as mentioned in the treatment of acute conditions). Much more effort has to be placed on the distal point stimulation in chronic spinal conditions. In some cases it is necessary to stimulate the point for up to 5 minutes. The point is stimulated until there is an appreciable warmth built up under the finger that does not disappear when the stimulation has stopped. As mentioned before, it is essential to create Ch'i in order to help and support the chronic lesion. Simply placing two fingers on the spine will not do anything. Success has to be worked for!!

Balancing Ch'i through the lesion

It is essential that Ch'i energy is stimulated at the site of the lesion. Unlike the acute lesion where the two points are merely held to create an energy flow, in chronic conditions the two points have to be stimulated first before they are held still. The pattern is to stimulate for up to 1 minute and then hold for a few seconds to see if there is a balance (sameness of sensation under the finger pads), then stimulate again for a few seconds, followed by a hold – and so on. In very chronic lesions this could take a few minutes, but stick at it; without creating an energy flow, nothing will happen and no results will be achieved!

Balancing the lesion site with the distal point

Once there is energy to work with, place the middle finger pad of one hand onto the most painful part of the lesion. This is not as easy as it may sound, because in chronic conditions there are several painful points. The therapist has to take into consideration the lesion diagnosis and the extent of the painful area before the exact lesion site is isolated. This stage of the procedure is one of the most important to perform correctly. It is important that a change of emphasis takes place under the fingers (8 Hz achieved). It is only then that true healing can take place.

Balance lesion site with associated reflexes

1. *Parallel zone.* The parallel zone obviously lies on the same vertical zone as the lesion area – the spine. The importance of the Lovett brother association was discussed in Chapter 5. In practice, it is necessary to place the hand (or relevent fingers) into the lesion area and the other hand over the Lovett brother association. The direction of angulation in the different areas of the spine is important in practice, and this will be discussed in specific spinal level treatment later in the chapter. It is possible to use the Lovett brother reflected area as the points for unwinding at the end of the treatment.
2. *Foot and hand.* These reflected points have been discussed several times before. The foot reflex appears to be the more powerful of the two, hence it is used much more by therapists. Do not,

however, dismiss the hand reflex as being insignificant; it isn't. The hand reflex can be of the utmost importance in the treatment of acutely painful aspects of chronic conditions.

3. *Ear.* The ear reflexes are often overlooked in acupressure; they seem to be much more popular when using acupuncture. More should be made of the ear reflexes, especially when there is a great deal of pain associated with the lesion. The reflected area in the ear will always be raised, slightly puffy and tender to the touch. On no account try to bore a hole in the ear; as with all reflected points, treat it with due care and consideration. The little finger is probably the best digit to use, as it is the most convenient to fit onto the very small reflex. The reflex should be given gentle stimulation followed by balancing between the ear and the lesion. Often this balance has to be held for up to 3–4 minutes.

4. *Stretch reflexes of the skull.* The great beauty of these little-known reflected points and areas is that they are very effective when there is a great deal of muscle spasm present. Once the correct reflex has been located (remember that there is not much tenderness with these), the extremities of the reflex need to be gently stretched apart, thus building up heat in the area. After about 2 minutes of doing this, the local area on the skull will be warm and the patient will inform the therapist that there is an increase of warmth and relaxation in the lesion area. There is no need to balance the skull reflex with the lesion.

Mobilization and manipulation

The therapist should never lose track of original skills. These include the capability to mobilize and possibly manipulate the offending vertebra. All the preceding acupressure performed on the spine will mean that the vertebra will be much more receptive to being adjusted, if it needs adjustment. There will be far less tissue trauma and the recovery rate of the patient will be quicker than if the vertebra is adjusted 'cold'. In chronic long-standing conditions the manipulative force needed to adjust the vertebra correctly will naturally be more than in acute conditions, but this does not mean that thrust techniques need be used – they are rarely employed. With the patient comfortable, place a couple of fingers onto the spasm (weak) side of the vertebra to be adjusted and hold the spasm until it starts to 'melt' away – this may take up to 2 minutes. A rotational or sideways adjustment should now be very easy to perform. Try to utilize the patient's natural forces and get him or her to assist you whenever possible – for example, make use of the weight of the patient's head when adjusting a cervical vertebra.

Unwinding the lesion

This technique is exactly the same as that discussed in the treatment of peripheral joint conditions and acute spinal lesions. The only difference with chronic spinal conditions is that the unwinding of the muscles and ligaments will be a lot slower than when dealing with acute conditions. There are three ways to unwind the lesion, depending on where it is:

1. The most used and possibly most effective way to unwind is to place both hands gently either side of the lesion, first on the spine just proximal and distal to the lesion and secondly either side of the spine. Each unwinding may take up to 4–5 minutes. The patient will only unwind (the therapist is just the facilitator) to the level that he or she is capable of in that particular treatment session. There is no way that complete unwinding of a 35-year-old lesion will take place in the first treatment session.
2. Place the hands on the spine, with one hand over the lesion site and the other hand over the Lovett brother association. This can be a bit slower than the first method, but is equally as effective. Both types can be tried in one treatment session if required.
3. Place two or three fingers bilateral to the spine, with one set of fingers in the muscle spasm and the other fingers on the opposite side of the spinous process. In cervical lesions this is done with the patient lying supine, and in thoracic and lumbo-sacral lesions it is done with the patient prone. The fingers on the spasm side will soon become warm and start to free up the lesion, whilst the other fingers will be drawn towards the lesion. Remember it is essential to go with the movement and not to oppose it! After a couple of minutes and quite a lot of movement a 'still point' will be produced, where no movement takes place for quite a number of seconds. There will then follow a sudden movement away from the lesion site as the localized ligaments unwind. This procedure can be extremely effective.

Final balancing

The final energy balance of the treatment session is used as part of the treatment procedure and as a diagnostic confirmation of what has been achieved in that particular session. Powerful points on the governor channel that are proximal and distal to the lesion are used for this purpose. Specific points will be enumerated when discussing individual conditions later in the chapter. Either use both hands with the centres of the palms placed over the points, or place the pads of the middle fingers on the points. An energy balance should be achieved fairly quickly due to all the previous work done in the session. Once a balance is achieved, the hands or fingers should be kept in position until an energy shift is achieved. This will create harmony in the area. When used as a diagnostic tool, the final energy balance can be compared to a balance achieved either at the beginning of the treatment or at the end of the previous treatment, with comparatives recorded in the patient's notes.

Treatment of specific-level chronic spinal lesions

For the following examples of spinal lesions, the spine has been divided up into six sections. The various points used are the same for each vertebra within a particular section. The major difference is, of course, the symptomatology existing at each level. It is not possible to 'cure' a longstanding spinal condition in one treatment; therefore the outlines illustrated below will have to be repeated at each visit although, as the condition improves, a shortcut in treatment procedure can be carried out in subsequent visits. The main principle of treatment of a chronic lesion is to attempt to convert the chronic lesion into an acute one. This is very much easier to treat. The chronic lesions that can be treated with clinical acupressure are varied. They include spondylitis, spondylosis, prolapsed intervertebral disc lesions, subluxation and fixation of apophyseal joints, osteoarthritic changes, fibrositis and lumbago. In each of the following cases it is assumed that the leg length differential has already been adjusted.

Cervical spine, C1–C4

Areas covered and symptomatology

- Atlanto-occipital (C0–C1). This region of the spine is significant in that lesions associated with it can produce the most chronic conditions, not only incorporating pain and discomfort but all manner of altered sensations. This area affects the vagus nerve, and so any impingement to nerves and soft tissue at this spinal level can have far-reaching affects. This spinal level is responsible for part of the blood supply to the head (via the vertebral arteries), the inner ear, the brain and the autonomic nervous system (via the vagus nerve). Symptomatology includes headaches, migraine, high and low blood pressure, nervousness and anxiety, amnesia and other sleeping disorders, chronic tiredness, dizziness, vertigo, depression and light-headedness.
- Atlanto-axial (C1–C2). The areas covered are the eyes, ears, frontal sinuses, mastoid, tongue and forehead. Symptomatology includes sinus pain, gritty and tired eyes, earache, vertigo, fainting spells and high and low blood pressure. There is still a vagus nerve influence at this level, and lesions here are of the most traumatic – for example, whiplash injury with torn vertebral ligaments and subluxation of the apophyseal joint can lead to wide-ranging symptoms affecting the vagus nerve, such as stomach tension, kidney imbalance etc.
- C2–C3. Areas covered are the cheeks, outer ear, facial bones and some of the teeth (upper jaw). Symptoms include earache, gritty eyes, mastoid sinus pain, headaches and neuralgia.
- C3–C4. Areas covered are the nose, lips, lower jaw, cervical glands and Eustachian tube. The symptoms are enlarged adenoids and tonsillitis, hardness of hearing, catarrh, swollen glands and certain allergic responses. This vertebral level is said to be the pivotal joint of the cervical spine, and is very important in postural imbalance of the neck. It is also traditionally related to conditions of the rheumatoid type, and acupuncturists are taught to needle the special point in between the spinous processes of C3–C4 in combination with the key points of the eight extraordinary meridians in all cases of rheumatoid conditions.
- C4–C5. Areas covered are the throat, vocal chords, cervical

glands and pharynx. Symptoms are laryngitis, hoarseness and general throat conditions, including 'lump' sensations. All the preceding areas of the neck also exhibit local pain and inflammatory symptoms.

Treatment

1. Massage the painful local points plus the bladder meridian (there are no specific bladder meridian acupoints in this region except Bl 10). Next, massage the neuro-lymphatic regions shown in Figure 8.4, namely underneath the clavicles, across the anterior aspect of the shoulder and down the sternum. On the posterior aspect of the neck they are situated between the transverse processes. It is more than likely that these points will already have

Figure 8.4 Points used in the treatment of chronic lesions of C1, C2, C3, C4.

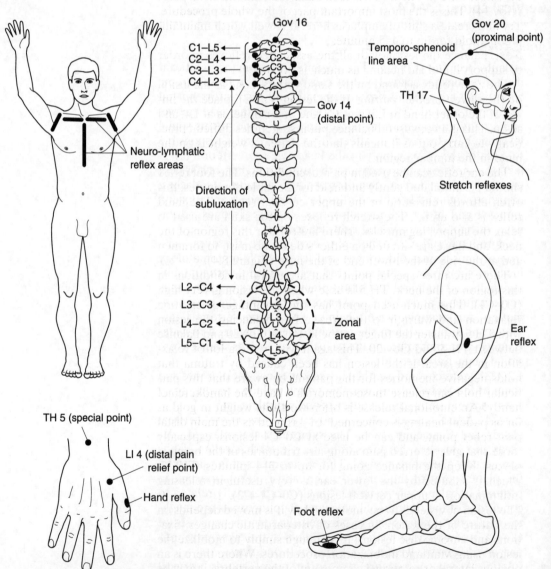

been stimulated, because they lie on the inner bladder line. These areas are painful and the patient should be warned of this in advance.

2. The distal point used to create energy is Gov 14, which is situated between the spinous processes of C7 and T1. This should be stimulated for up to 1 minute – or even longer – until an appreciable amount of heat is felt under the finger. It is essential that this part of the procedure is not hurried in order to pass quickly onto the next stage. Ch'i must be created in order to heal!!

3. The proximal point used for lesions in this area is Gov 20 (on top of the head). This point is stimulated slightly before balancing it with Gov 14. This now balances Ch'i energy through the lesion.

4. Now find the most painful part of the lesion (usually over the transverse process, but not always), and place the pad of the middle finger onto it. The lesion is then balanced with the distal point (Gov 14). This is the most important part of the whole procedure. Try and create a shift of emphasis here. It is well worth maintaining the hold for up to 4–5 minutes!

5. Next, balance the lesion with all the associated reflexes in order to support it and aid healing as much as possible:

    The zone reflex is found on the same vertical zone as the lesion on the Lovett brother pairing. If the lesion is at C1, place the finger of the other hand at L5; if at C2, the other finger is at L4, and so on. This is a very useful balance but is sometimes difficult practically to carry out as it means that the patient's weight is on the hand in the lumbar region.

    The ear reflex can be used in painful conditions. The foot reflex should be stimulated gently and held for a couple of minutes, this often affords relaxation in the upper cervical region. The hand reflex is also useful. The stretch reflexes on the skull are used to relax the supporting muscles. There are two for this region of the neck, and these are situated on either side of the mastoid foramen and at the side of the lower end of the nose (Figure 8.4).

    There are three special points that are useful in conditions in this region of the neck. TH 5 is used when the lesion is very high (C0–C1). This much-used point has the advantage of creating relaxation and warmth to the area. After balancing the lesion with TH 5, transfer the finger on the lesion to Gov 20 and balance between TH 5 and Gov 20. This again will create a lot of relaxation in the area. If the lesion has been caused by trauma that holds negative memories for the patient, be aware that this particular hold can release those memories – have the handkerchief handy! An emotional release is often worth its weight in gold as far as patient healing is concerned. LI 4 is used as the main distal pain relief point, and can be used at C0–C4 lesions, especially those that give referred pain along any tributaries of the brachial plexus. Keep the balance going for up to 3–4 minutes. TH 17, which is situated by the lower ear, is very useful in releasing inflammation in upper cervical lesions (C0–C1–C2).

6. The lesion now needs to be 'moved'. How it is moved depends on the nature of the lesion. In cases of osteoarthritic changes, fixations and chronic disc lesions, it is enough simply to mobilize the lesion using Maitland mobilization procedures. Where there is an obvious lateral or rotational component of the vertebra, it may be

necessary to adjust. This has been described previously. It is essential that the adjacent vertebrae are also mobilized.

7. Unwinding is necessary to allow the congestion and spasm in the paravertebral muscles and ligaments to relax and to aid the alignment of the vertebra. Unwinding, as previously described, can be performed with the hands placed just superior and inferior to the lesion or with fingers placed either side. Another good way of unwinding is to place one hand over the lesion area and the other one over the associated Lovett brother. In this case, the hand is placed over L2–L5. There could be a considerable amount of unwinding taking place over a period of about 3–4 minutes. The torsion strain with unwinding will pull both hands towards the lesion side because the direction of the lesion, if there is lateral deviation, is towards the same side.

8. The final energy balance can incorporate the previous hold. It is also a good idea to balance between Gov 20 and Gov 14.

Cervical spine C5, C6, C7–T1

Areas covered and symptomatology

C5–C6. Areas covered are the base of the throat and upper bronchus, shoulders and the lower neck. Symptoms are stiff and painful neck, pain in shoulder and upper forearm, croup, tonsillitis and bronchitis.

C6–C7. Areas covered are the thyroid gland, shoulders, elbows and medial side of the hand. Symptoms include thyroid conditions, proneness to catching colds.

C7–T1. Areas covered are the forearms and the lateral aspect of the hand, the oesophagus, trachea and the upper medial aspect of the chest. Symptoms include throat conditions, mild asthma and referred pain along the brachial plexus, including parasthesia. This is a most significant vertebral level, and is commonly called the cervico-thoracic junction. It seems to be the centre of the parallelogram of forces that act vertically up and down the spine and bilaterally across to the shoulders. This level is therefore prone to a great deal of stress and tension. In esoteric terms it represents the posterior aspect of the throat chakra.

T1–T2. Areas covered are the upper aspect of the heart including the coronory arteries. Symptoms include heart conditions, some forms of chest pain, angina and pain in the little finger. The energy flow from this level governs bone. As mentioned before, it is used in any condition of osteoarthritic change and discontinuity of bone. It seems to have an energic relationship to the parathyroids.

Treatment

1. Massage the local acupoints, together with the inner bladder line. Along this line are the posterior points of the neuro-lymphatic reflexes. The anterior reflexes are shown in Figure 8.5, and are found underneath the clavicles, across the anterior aspect of the shoulder and either side of the sternum. Deep massage is

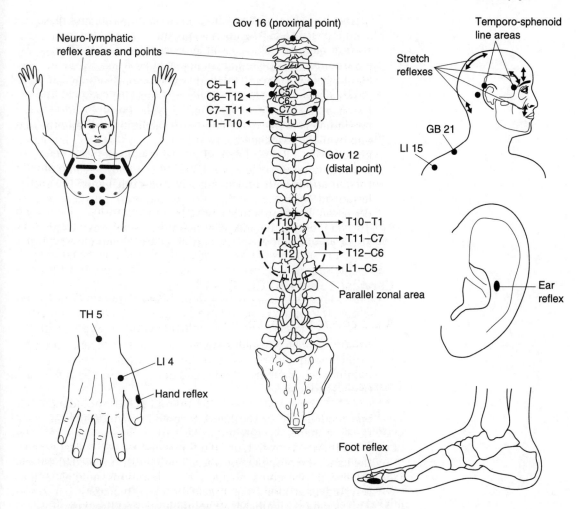

Figure 8.5 Points used in the treatment of chronic lesions of C5, C6, C7, T1.

extremely important with lesions in this area. There is often some fibrositis present, or painful fibromyalgia. Connective tissue massage is the massage of choice in the initial stages of the treatment. Do not hurry the initial massage, it is vitally important.

2. The best distal point is Gov 12, which is situated between the spinous processes of T2 and T3. This point should be stimulated for up to 2 minutes, especially in long-standing stress conditions.

3. The proximal point is Gov 16, situated between the occiput and the atlas. This point should be stimulated for a few seconds and then energy balanced with Gov 12 so as to allow an energy flow through the lesion.

4. Next, place the pad of the middle finger on the lesion. This is now balanced with Gov 12. Again, it is emphasized that the energy balancing between the lesion and the distal point is the most important part of the treatment. Take care that it is not hurried.

5. Now balance the lesion with the associated reflex and special points. The zone reflex is situated between T10 and L1, which is the same as the Lovett brother. The hand, foot and ear reflexes can be used, especially where there is much pain. The foot reflex is particularly effective for stress and tension around the cervico-thoracic

junction. There are six stretch reflexes on the skull, and these are shown in Figure 8.5. The main one is situated over the eyes – give a vertical pull above the eyes at approximately GB 14. Two of the special points are the same as for upper cervical lesions, namely TH 5 and LI 4. There are two other very useful points situated at LI 15 and GB 21. LI 15 is very good when treating stress around the cervico-thoracic junction. Balancing between the lesion and LI 15 should be done over a period of at least 2 minutes in order to gain the maximum advantage.

6.   The vertebrae can now be mobilized or manipulated according to the type of lesion. Even if the vertebra is manipulated, it should always be mobilized immediately afterwards, together with the adjacent vertebrae.

7.   Unwinding is best done with the patient lying prone, placing one hand over the lesion area and the other hand over the Lovett brother association of T10–L1. Whilst unwinding, remember that the torsion strains will be opposite to each other as the lateral pull is in the opposite direction. Unwinding will improve with practice!!

8.   Final energy balancing is best done between points Gov 16 and the Lovett brother, so as to have the lesion area between the two hands. This should be done with the patient lying supine with the therapist's hands placed underneath.

Thoracic spine

The whole of the thoracic spine has been 'lumped together' here because the order of treatment is exactly the same at each level. The only differences that exist with each individual vertebra are the positioning on the temporo-sphenoidal line in the initial analysis and the symptomatology occurring at each level. The thoracic spine represents a large field on the temporo-sphenoidal line (Figure 3.15), and it is relatively easy (with practice) to discern between, say, a T3 lesion and one at T5.

Areas covered and symptomatology

- T2, T3, T4. This double vertebral complex is the main level for treatment of the lungs, bronchii, pleurae, chest and mammary glands. The symptoms are most chest conditions, including bronchitis, pleurisy and lung congestion; also chest pains (unless there is a nerve referral from the brachial plexus), mastitis and conditions that affect the lymphatic supply to the breast tissue.

- T4–T5. The areas covered are the gall bladder and the hepatic duct, giving symptoms associated with gall bladder colic, indigestion, jaundice and some types of shingles.

- T5–T6. This level governs the liver, solar plexus and diaphragm, giving symptoms of tension in the diaphragm, liver conditions, fevers, low blood pressure, anaemia and poor circulation. The latter is because there is also a deep energetic flow to the heart and the pericardium. Anatomically this vertebral level is extremely important, as it represents the pivotal region of the spine. The Lovett brother of T5 is T6. In practical terms, this means that scoliosis is often found specifically at this level due to previous spinal postural imbalances. It is often said that the whole spine 'revolves' around T5–T6, and to have a strong, supported vertebra here means, generally, a healthy individual.

- T6–T7. The area covered is the stomach, giving symptoms concerned with that organ. These include gastritis, ulcers, 'nervous' stomach, indigestion, heartburn and dyspepsia.
- T7–T8. Areas covered are the pancreas and duodenum, giving symptoms related to diabetes, duodenal ulcers and general tension in the diaphragmatic region.
- T8–T9. Areas covered are the spleen and, again, the diaphragm. This gives rise to symptoms associated with the spleen, such as altered auto-immune conditions (e.g. chronic fatigue syndrome). Other symptoms include general lethargy and hiccoughs.
- T9–T10. The adrenals and suprarenals are covered by this vertebral level. The symptoms of imbalance include lowered immune response, hyper- or hypo-adrenia or general lack of production of cortisone. Many allergies can occur due to imbalance at this level. There is also an energetic supply to the liver, hence the influence on allergies.
- T10–T11. The kidneys are associated with this level, giving symptoms of kidney conditions, chronic tiredness, nephritis and pyelitis.
- T11–T12. Areas covered are the kidney with the ureters. Symptoms include those of the previous level, plus some skin conditions such as acne, eczema and boils.
- T12–L1. The areas covered by this level are the ileum and the jejunal region of the small bowel, and the Fallopian tubes. Symptoms may include those of irritable bowel syndrome, generalized gut flora imbalance and bowel inflammation; also certain types of sterility.

Treatment

1. Massage the local points on the thoracic spine. It is easy to combine massaging the inner bladder meridian points and the posterior neuro-lymphatic points because they all appear on the same line but at different depths. The best way to massage down the thoracic spine is to place the index finger and middle finger either side of a vertebra at the level of the transverse processes and stimulate each point for a few seconds before going on to the next level. The whole of the thoracic spine can then be given stimulating massage with several sweeps in a few seconds. The anterior neuro-lymphatic points are positioned either side of the sternum and underneath the costal angle of the lower ribs. This latter area is specifically associated with tension in the thoracic spine, as well as being the neuro-lymphatic area to the quadriceps group of muscles.
2. The distal point to create energy is Gov 3, which is situated between the spinous processes of L4–L5 (Figure 8.6). In most chronic thoracic lesions this point has to be stimulated for up to 3–4 minutes before an appreciable change of sensation is felt under the finger.
3. The proximal point is Gov 14 (C7–T1), and the proximal and distal points are now stimulated together and then the points held in

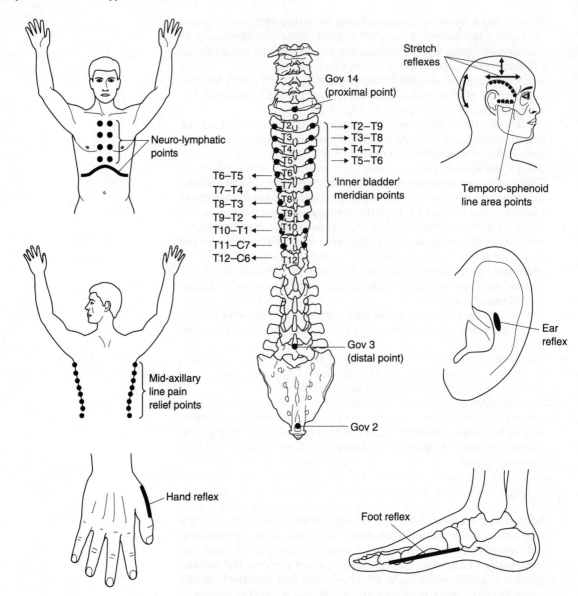

Figure 8.6   Points used in the treatment of chronic lesions of the thoracic spine.

order to create a balance of energy and a flow of energy through the thoracic spine.

4.   Now find the specific lesion area and balance it with Gov 3. As has been stated on numerous occasions, this is the most important aspect of the treatment and needs to be done with care. Make sure there is an energy shift during this phase.

5.   The lesion now needs to be balanced with all its associated reflexes. The foot reflexes are usually very tender (especially where there are any symptoms concerning the diaphragm and the spleen); the hand reflex is also useful and can be used as a home exercise for the patient. The ear reflex is particularly good when there is very acute pain. The best reflexes, though, appear down the mid-axillary line. A tender point will be found in the mid-axillary line situated on the same intercostal level as the lesion. The

balance between the lesion and this pain relief reflex is very effective! After this hold has been completed, it may be opportune to use the associated stretch reflexes on the skull. The advantage of using these is to reduce muscle tension, which nearly always exists in chronic lesions at this level. Do not use the Lovett brother association at this point, because it will be used later in the unwinding.

6. Now is the time to mobilize or manipulate the lesion. Thoracic spine lesions answer very well to transverse process stretching and Maitland mobilizing. Do not forget to mobilize the rib facets as well as the vertebra.

7. Unwinding the area by placing one hand over the lesion and the other hand over the Lovett brother. If these points are close together, e.g. T5 and T6, then it is obvious that unwinding has to be done with fingers *in situ* and not the whole hand. Also be aware that there will be an opposite direction torsion strain as the lesion unwinds.

8. The final energy balance is done between the original distal and proximal points of Gov 3 and Gov 14. The therapist will find that the balance is achieved much more quickly at this stage than at the beginning of the treatment. It is sometimes necessary to substitute Gov 2 (sacro-coccyx) for Gov 3 as the distal point in some very long-standing lesions, especially when there is much scoliosis of the spine.

Lumbar spine, L1, L2, L3

Although the lumbar vertebrae are much larger anatomically than the cervical and thoracic vertebrae, and play a different role in the supporting structure of the spine, it is far easier to ascertain a specific thoracic lesion than a specific lumbar one. This is due to several factors. When there is a chronic lesion of the lumbar spine, this is accompanied by gross muscle spasm, weakness, lymphatic congestion, pain (both local and referred), deformity and postural changes. It is not helped by the area of the temporo-sphenoidal line associated with the lumbar spine being small; hence it is not an easy task to delineate between, say, an L1 and an L2 lesion. Even the areas covered and the symptomatology are similar. As every professional therapist knows, the lower lumbar region is much more prone to conditions related to wear and tear and old postural changes. The upper lumbar spine, which is covered in this section, is not so affected by weight-bearing and old postural problems.

Areas covered and symptomatology

- L1–L2. The areas covered are the bulk of the large bowel and the inguinal cavity of the groin. This can give rise to the following symptoms when there is an imbalance at this level; constipation, colitis, diarrhoea and hernia pain. Lesions at this level also affect what is traditionally called the 'lower heater'. This means that some lesions at this level can produce coldness in the loins, lower spine and legs, causing circulatory conditions such as chilblains and cold feet.

- L2–L3. The areas covered are the appendix region (including the ileo-caecal valve), the upper aspect of the leg and the lower abdomen. Symptoms include those of appendicitis (very common!!) and ileo-caecal valve syndrome, general cramps in the abdomen and alternating constipation and diarrhoea. Lesions at this level can also give rise to chronic tiredness and sluggishness elimination of urine.
- L3–L4. Areas covered are the sex organs and the bladder. There is also a referral to the knee area. Symptoms include bladder conditions, menstrual conditions such as painful and irregular periods, menopausal symptoms, bed-wetting, and many knee conditions.

Figure 8.7 Points used in the treatment of chronic lesions of L1, L2, L3.

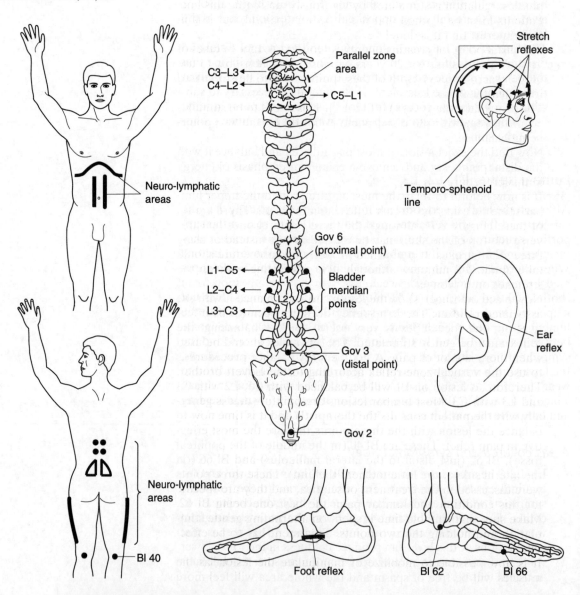

Treatment

1.   Massage the local points around and including the lesion area. This will include meridian (bladder) and non-meridian points. Also massage the neuro-lymphatic areas associated with the upper lumbar area. These are situated posteriorly locally around the upper lumbar region and in a triangle shape around the lower lumbar area (Figure 8.7). Anteriorly, they are on the lower costal margin and bilaterally on the median line of the abdomen area. There is also an important area on the ilio-tibial tract. This area was mentioned fully in the acute spinal lesion section. Suffice it to say, when dealing with chronic lumbar lesions this region has much more significance. In every case of a chronic lumbo-sacral lesion, there is always lymphatic circulation congestion. The lymphatic circulation is stimulated by vigorously massaging this line. Patients must be warned that it can be very painful, but it is in their interest that it is done!

2.   The distal point for creating energy is Gov 3 (L4–L5). In cases of very chronic lesions (of 20 years or more) it is advisable to use Gov 2 (sacro-coccyx). Both of these points have to be stimulated for at least 2–3 minutes.

3.   The proximal point is Gov 6 (T12–L1). This needs to be stimulated in tandem with the distal point, followed by the two points being balanced.

4.   Now find the exact lesion or most painful area and balance it with the distal point. Try and achieve a change of emphasis of energy in this procedure.

5.   It is now helpful to relax the musculature around the upper lumbar spine by using the stretch reflexes on the skull. There are six of these (Figure 8.7), although the three bilateral ones that traverse the top of the skull may be treated as one instead of using three short strokes. If performed properly this procedure should take about 2–3 minutes, although it is comforting to keep the stretches on for longer.

6.   Now place the finger(s) on the lesion site and balance it with the associated reflexes. The hand reflex does not seem to be effective, but the foot reflex is very useful. Before balancing, the reflex must be gently stimulated. The ear reflex should be used when there is a lot of pain. A good energy balance procedure is to use the vertical zone reflex according to the Lovett brother. Therefore, a lesion on L1 will be balanced with C5, L2 with C4 and L3 with C3. Most lumbar lesions are painful (that is generally why the patient consults the therapist!) and it is time now to balance the lesion with the three points that are the most effective in pain relief. These are Bl 40 (in the middle of the popliteal fossa), Bl 62 (just distal to the lateral malleolus) and Bl 66 (on the lateral side of the little toe near the end). These three points were discussed in the treatment of sciatica, and they are specific for this condition and lumbar pain, the best one being Bl 62. Make sure that suitable time is spent on alternating gentle stimulation and holding the two points. Treatment has to be effective!!

7.   It is now possible to mobilize or manipulate the lesion, as the muscles will be free of spasm and the whole area will feel more

comfortable. It is important not to create more pain and protective spasm in the act of manipulation, so be gentle!
8. Unwind the area by placing one hand over the lower lumbar spine and the other hand over the parallel area zone between C3 and C5.
9. Final energy balancing is done between the proximal and distal points, as used at the beginning of the treatment.

Lumbar spine, L4, L5, S1

This region of the spine is the one that takes most of the body weight, and it is therefore subject to more strain than any other part of the body. It is no surprise then to find that physiotherapists, osteopaths, chiropractors, masseurs etc. spend more person-hours in treating this anatomical region than any other. Treating chronic low back conditions with clinical acupressure can be very rewarding. Experience has shown that the time factor of patient recovery is less than when treating with other modalities. There is also the added bonus that there is far less treatment trauma for the patient to endure!

Areas covered and symptomatology

- L4–L5. Areas covered by nerves from this level are the prostate gland, muscles of the lower back and the upper part of the sciatic nerve. This gives the following symptoms; sciatica, lumbago, difficult or painful urination and backache. There is also a deep energy flow through to the large bowel, which often gives rise to sluggishness of the bowel.
- L5–S1. Areas covered are the lower limbs, middle part of the sciatic nerve, ankles, feet and toes. Symptoms of imbalance are poor circulation in the legs, swollen ankles, weak ankles and arches, cold feet, weakness in the legs, cramps and sciatica. The energy flow is to the small bowel, and imbalance at this level can cause irritable bowel syndrome and ulceration in long-standing low back pain.

Treatment

1. Massage the local points. These are normally the bladder points that lie between the transverse processes. Also massage the neuro-lymphatic points and areas; these lie either side of the spine at the level of the lesion, at the sacro-iliac joints, the ilio-tibial tract, the lateral aspect of the calves and a small area on the medial aspect of the knee (around Li 8). Anteriorly, the areas lie down the anterior aspect of the lower abdomen. Make sure that the patient realizes that these points and areas are painful. It is best to massage them with oil.
2. The distal point that is stimulated to create energy is Gov 2 (sacro-coccyx). In very long-standing lesions, the stimulation can often take 4–5 minutes! It is also comforting to the patient to rest the other hand on the lower lumbar spine whilst this point is being stimulated. It can be off-putting for patients to have this area stimulated if the reason for doing so is not fully explained to them.

3. The proximal point is at Gov 6 (T12–L1). Stimulate this point and then balance it with Gov 2 to allow energy to flow through the lesion.
4. Place a finger pad on the lesion and leave it there for a few seconds. Now balance it with Gov 2. This balance is the most crucial part of the treatment, and there should be a shift of emphasis whilst doing it. The whole area will now feel much more comfortable and less painful.
5. The lesion is now balanced with the associated reflected points. The foot reflex should be stimulated for a few seconds before balancing it with the lesion. Next, balance the lesion with bladder points down the leg. These are at Bl 40 (posterior aspect of popliteal fossa), Bl 62 (underneath the lateral malleolus) and Bl 66 (lateral aspect of the little toe). Each balance should take a couple of minutes. These points are useful where there is a lot of pain, but are of extra special use when there is sciatica. Now stretch the scalp reflexes – there are three areas (Figure 8.8). The

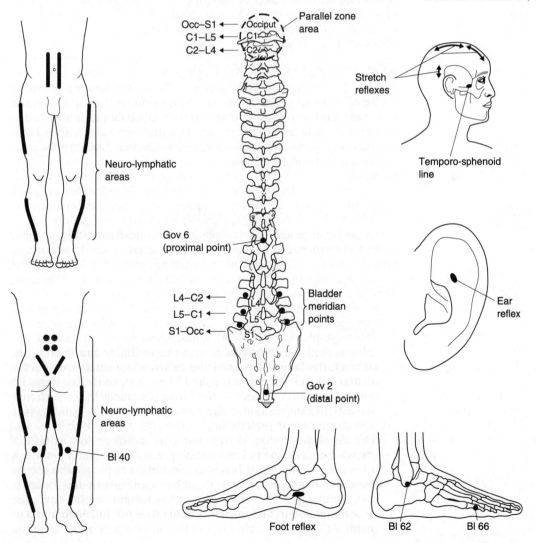

Figure 8.8 Points used in the treatment of chronic lesions of L4, L5, S1.

ear reflex point can also be massaged. This is particularly good when there is a lot of soreness in the area.

6. It is now time to mobilize or manipulate the region. Experience shows that the majority of chronic low back problems are due to old injuries that create a fixation at the apophyseal joints. These answer superbly to Maitland mobilizing as well as lateral or rotational stretches up to Grade V. Genuine prolapsed intervertebral disc lesions are comparatively rare!!

7. Unwind the area by placing one hand over the sacrum and the other hand on the upper cervical region. This area is also the Lovett brother. There is often a compensatory lesion of the upper cervical spine that side-shifts in the same direction as the lower lumbar lesion. Therefore, when unwinding the supporting muscles, expect that there will be a torsion strain, with both hands pulling towards the same side until the release occurs.

8. The final energy balance is done between Gov 2 and Gov 6. The balance of energy will be achieved much more quickly than at the beginning of the treatment!

Sacrum and coccyx

As has been stated before, the sacrum can be represented as the foundation of a building, the remainder of the vertebra being the other floors. It is therefore imperative to have a stable foundation, otherwise the other floors will become out of alignment and mechanical lesions will ensue. It is essential when treating any chronic spinal condition, even upper cervical ones, that the sacrum is treated for pain, stiffness and malalignment and is also energy balanced with the cranium!

Areas covered and symptomatology

The areas covered are those supplied by the lower aspect of the sciatic nerve and sacral plexus, the hips, buttocks, rectum, anus and sex organs. Some symptoms that occur due to imbalance within the sacrum/coccyx are sacro-iliitis, sacro-iliac subluxation and fixation, spinal scoliosis, sciatica, haemorrhoids, pruritis, coccydinia and foot pain.

Treatment

1. Massage all the local bladder points, including the ones in the sacral foramen and the ones that lie over the sacro-iliac joints. It is worth the effort of spending a few seconds on stimulating each one in turn. Stimulating or connective tissue massage will already have been performed, so the tissues should be relatively warm and the patient may not grimace with such pain as if the area had not been massaged beforehand. Also massage the associated neuro-lymphatic points and areas. These are situated posteriorly along the sacro-iliac joints, the ilio-tibial tracts and the medial aspect of the shins. Anteriorly, they lie on the medial aspect of the upper leg and around Li 8 on the medial aspect of the knee. It is also useful to massage the whole length of the bladder meridian from the lower back down to the outer aspect of the little toe.

2. The distal point to create energy is either Gov 2 (sacro-coccyx) if it is predominantly a sacral lesion or Gov 1 (tip of coccyx) if it is a coccyx lesion (Figure 8.9). However, massaging Gov 1 can have severe drawbacks due to its anatomy! If the therapist thinks that it is prudent to stimulate it, make sure there is a chaperone in the room! An excellent alternating distal point is Li 8 (on the medial aspect of the knee joint). This point will always be tender in any sacro-coccygeal lesion, so take care when stimulating it. Incidentally, Li 8 is also a specific acupressure point in the treatment of cold feet, so there may be an added bonus when treating some patients.

3. The proximal point is Gov 3 (L4–L5). Make sure that this point is stimulated and then energy balanced with the distal point in order to create an energy flow through the area.

Figure 8.9 Points used in the treatment of chronic sacrum and coccyx conditions.

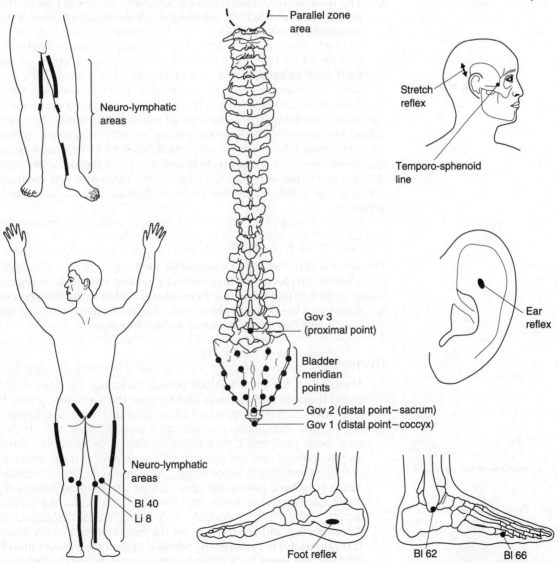

4.   Now find the lesion (whichever is the most painful or sluggish point) and balance it with the distal point. This procedure has to be prolonged to ensure that a change of energy emphasis is made.

5.   Next, balance the lesion with the various associated reflexes. The foot reflex can be stimulated and then balanced with the lesion. If there is much leg pain, the lesion can be balanced with Bl 40, Bl 62 and Bl 66, as described in the previous section. This should ease most sciatic referrals. The most effective energy balancing with the sacrum, however, is with the zones. The topic of cranio-sacral reflexology was discussed in Chapter 5, and Figure 5.2 shows a chart of the various vertical and horizontal zones of the sacrum. In chronic lesions of the sacrum, these zone reflexes may be used in two ways. If the lesion (painful point) lies on the superior aspect of the sacrum, balance it with the same vertical zone point on the occiput. Make sure that each point is held with the pads of the two middle fingers. If the lesion lies on the sacro-iliac joint, place one finger on the painful point and the whole hand on the associated zone on the spine – for example, if the tender point lies on Zone 4 of the sacrum, place one finger on the painful point and the other hand first on the L3–4 level and secondly on the C4–6 level, both these spinal levels being Zone 4 areas. This may sound complicated at first, but in practice it is relatively easy. Taking the hand away from the lesion, the ear reflex needs to be stimulated and the scalp reflex also needs to be treated. Next, the whole hand should be placed on the sacrum (it is usually more comfortable to place the hand with the heel of the hand at the lower edge and the fingers pointing upwards) and the other hand placed on the base of the occiput. This procedure can be done with the patient lying either prone or supine. Each position has its merits and drawbacks.

6.   Mobilization can now be carried out using whatever method the therapist is trained in. It is not usually necessary to use a lot of force if the sacro-iliac joint needs adjusting; the area will be so relaxed that very little force should be needed.

7.   The sacrum/coccyx is unwound by placing one hand vertically over the area and the other hand over the base of the skull, as per the Lovett brother correspondence. If the therapist feels that the lesion will benefit from using a different area to unwind (this depends on the cause), then the sacrum can be unwound with any other part of the vertebral column.

8.   The final energy balance is done between Gov 3 and either Gov 1/2 or Ki 1 on the sole of the foot.

References

Academy of Traditional Chinese Medicine (1975). *An Outline of Chinese Acupuncture*. Foreign Language Press.

Becker, R. (1976). Electrophysiological correlates of acupuncture points and meridians. *Psychoenergetic Systems,* **1**, 105–12.

Chang, C. Y. and Chang, C. T. (1973). Peripheral afferent pathway for acupuncture anaesthesia. *Scientica Sinica,* **16**, 210–17.

Chapman C. R. *et al.* (1997). Effects of intrasegmental electrical acupuncture on dental pain: evaluation by threshold estimation and sensory decision theory. *Pain,* **3**, 213–27.

Cross, J. (1986). *The Relationship of the Chakra Energy System and Acupuncture*. Doctoral Thesis. Copyright held by British College of Acupuncture.

Cross, J. (in preparation). *Healing with the Chakra Energy System*.

Ebner, M. (1962*). Connective Tissue Massage – Theory and Therapeutic Application*. E. & S. Livingstone Ltd.

Ellis, N. (1994). *Acupuncture in Clinical Practice*. Chapman and Hall.

Gach, M. R. (1990). *Acupressure – How to Cure Common Ailments the Natural Way*. Piatkus Publishing.

Gerber, R. (1988). *Vibrational Medicine – New Choices for Healing Ourselves*. Bear and Company.

Grinberg, A. (1989). *Holistic Reflexology*. Thorsons Publishing Group.

Hunt, V. (1995). *Infinite Mind*. Malibu Publishing Co.

Lawson-Wood, D. and Lawson-Wood, J. (1960). *Judo Revival Points, Athletes' Points and Posture*. Health Science Press.

Lazorthes, Y. (1990). Acupuncture meridians and radiotracers. *Pain,* **40**, 109–12.

Lewith, G. and Lewith, N. R. (1994). *Modern Chinese Acupuncture*, Chapter 5. Green Print.

Low, R. (1988). *The Non-Meridial Points of Acupuncture*. Thorsons Publishing Group.

Maitland, G. D. (1986). *Vertebral Manipulation* (5th edn). Butterworths.

Maxwell Cade, C. (1979). *The Awakened Mind* (1996 reprint). Element Books.

Melzack, R. (1977). Trigger points and acupuncture points for pain: correlations and implications. *Pain*, **3**, 3–23.

Mitchie, J. (1996). There is no evidence to support the existence of acupuncture points or meridians. *J. Acupuncture Assoc. Chartered Physiotherapists*, March.

Mochizuki, J. S. (1995). *Anma – the Art of Japanese Massage*. Kotobuki Publications.

Motoyama, H. (1988). *Theories of the Chakras – Bridge to Higher Consciousness*. Theosophical Publishing House.

Shrenberger, R. (1977). Acupuncture meridians retain their identity after death. *Am. J. Acupuncture*, **5(4)**, 357–61.

Stormer, C. (1995). *Reflexology – The Definitive Guide*. Hodder and Stoughton.

Sutherland, W. G. (1990). *Teachings in the Science of Osteopathy*. Rudra Press.

Thie, J. F. (1979). *Touch For Health – A New Approach to Restoring our Natural Energies*. DeVorss and Co.

Thompson, W.H. (1973). *Acupuncture – As Far as we Know*. The First Korth Lecture. Acupuncture Association and Register Ltd.

Thompson, W. H. (1985). *Personalised Diagnosis – Alternative Medicine*. Published privately.

Tiberiu, R. (1981) Do meridians and acupuncture points exist? A radioactive tracer study of the bladder. *Am. J. Acupuncture*, **9(3)**, 251–6.

Vernejoul, P. (1992). Nuclear medicine and acupuncture message transmission. *J. Nuclear Med.*, **33(3)**, 409–12.

Wagner, F. (1978). *Reflex Zone Massage – The Handbook of Therapy and Self-Help*. Thorsons Publishing Group.

Walther, D. S. (1976). *Applied Kinesiology – The Advanced Approach in Chiropractic*. Systems D.C.

Zong-Xiang, Z. (1981). Research advances in the electrical specificity of meridians and acupuncture points. *Am. J. Acupuncture*, **9(3)**, 203–16.

Index